NURSING TEAM LEADERSHIP

Second Edition

THORA KRON, R.N., B.S.
Consultant in Team Nursing; formerly Nurse-Director, Practical Nursing Program, Area Vocational-Technical School, Grand Rapids, Minnesota; formerly Clinical Instructor in Medical and Surgical Nursing, St. Luke's Hospital School of Nursing, Duluth, Minnesota

W. B. SAUNDERS COMPANY

Philadelphia and London

W. B. Saunders Company: West Washington Square,
                          Philadelphia, Pa. 19105

                          12 Dyott Street
                          London, W.C.1

Reprinted July, 1966, August, 1967, December, 1967 and December, 1968.

Nursing Team Leadership

© 1966 by W. B. Saunders Company. Copyright 1961 by W. B. Saunders Company. Copyright under the International Copyright Union. All rights reserved. This book is protected by copyright. No part of it may be duplicated or reproduced without written permission from the publisher. Made in the United States of America. Press of W. B. Saunders Company. Library of Congress catalog card number 66-12417.

To
Nursing
Team Leaders

Preface to the Second Edition

The objectives of this revision are (1) to bring the information up to date and (2) to include more information about those activities which, in the author's opinion, are important in the effective practice of team leadership.

Bibliographies have been brought up to date and some study questions have been revised. The section on changes in medicine and in nursing philosophy, education, and practice has been rewritten. New material has been added to the sections on supervision and communication, on the functions of the team leader and her team members, including the licensed practical nurse, on planning nursing care, and on the role of the head nurse in team nursing. A section on the legal responsibilities of the professional nurse as team leader has been added.

Professional nurses continue to ask, What is the role of the professional nurse? and How can we give nursing care to our patients? The author continues to feel that utilization of the concepts of the team plan is the only way that each nurse can find satisfactory answers to these questions.

This book is still directed toward helping the professional nursing student prepare for her role as team leader and giving the nurse who is unfamiliar with team nursing a simple guide to the effective practice of the concepts of team nursing. The author does not intend to provide an exhaustive dissertation or a profoundly intellectual approach to these concepts. The information included in this book provides the professional nurse with a starting point from which she should continue to increase her professional stature by discovering additional ways of applying these principles in her own situation.

The author wishes to thank the many professional nurses who offered helpful suggestions and criticisms during various workshops on team nursing and in professional meetings. Special acknowledgment is extended to Helen Hill Blanz, LL.B., for her help in writing the section on the legal responsibilities of the team leader.

Floodwood, Minnesota THORA KRON

Preface to the First Edition

The nursing profession needs more leaders—in administration, in education, and, perhaps more than ever before, in the giving of nursing care. Schools of nursing, recognizing this need, are gradually enlarging their curricula to include learning experiences designed to prepare the nursing student for assuming her place as a leader.

Some years ago industry and education began to realize the importance of good human relations and democratic leadership in producing better job performance. In nursing, the focal point has been, and always will be, the patient; however, the nurse who derives satisfaction from, and feels secure in, her work will be able to provide better care for the patient. Today the role of the nurse is changing from one who *gives* care to one who *directs* and *supervises* the care given by others. The nursing profession is also beginning to realize that the old concepts of autocratic supervision are less effective in providing good patient care than are the techniques of democratic leadership.

Team nursing was devised so that the professional nurse could make better use of her knowledge and skills by guiding others in the giving of nursing care. The techniques that the nurse must use in planning, directing, supervising, and evaluating the work of her team are based upon those principles used by a leader in any field. The experience gained as a team leader is an excellent way of preparing for leadership in any nursing endeavor. For this reason, every nurse, preferably while she is still a student, should have a thorough indoctrination in the principles of team nursing and in the techniques of team leadership.

In one school of nursing, whenever the students studied team nursing and their responsibilities as team leaders, they had difficulty in finding professional reference material relating to specific ways of carrying out the duties of a leader. Most of the available information was directed toward preparing the nurse for more advanced administrative or supervisory positions. In some areas, such as communications and human relations, the students had to adapt methods that were described for the use of industry. From this difficulty of finding sufficient material suitable for classroom use was born the idea of a book on leadership in nursing that would draw its information from many sources and adapt it for the use of the professional nurse, especially the nursing team leader.

This book was prepared primarily for nursing students or recent graduates who need a simple guide to use in increasing their effectiveness in team leadership; however, other professional nurses should find it worthwhile for reviewing the principles set down and illustrated herein. Many of the illustrations and suggestions included in this book grew out of classroom discussions in which the nursing students and their instructor explored together the concept of team nursing and the methods of practicing democratic team leadership. The author wishes to take this opportunity to acknowledge the contribution of these students.

The author also wishes to extend her appreciation to the many professional nurses and nurses' aides throughout the United States who provided essential information and helpful suggestions in answer to the various questionnaires. Grateful appreciation is also given to Mrs. Barbara Kurtz, who provided both information and encouragement, and to Mrs. Mary Cadigan, who assisted in building the bibliography for the manuscript.

Finally, special acknowledgment is given to Mrs. Alice Kohler, who, although she is unaware of it, contributed to making this book a reality through her devotion to nursing and her desire to improve nursing education.

Floodwood, Minnesota THORA KRON

Beatitudes of a Leader

Blessed is the leader who has not sought the high places, but who has been drafted into service because of his ability and willingness to serve.

Blessed is the leader who knows where he is going, why he is going, and how to get there.

Blessed is the leader who knows no discouragement, who presents no alibi.

Blessed is the leader who knows how to lead without being dictatorial; true leaders are humble.

Blessed is the leader who seeks for the best for those he serves.

Blessed is the leader who leads for the good of the most concerned, and not for the personal gratification of his own ideas.

Blessed is the leader who develops leaders while leading.

Blessed is the leader who marches with the group, interprets correctly the signs on the pathway that leads to success.

Blessed is the leader who has his head in the clouds but his feet on the ground.

Blessed is the leader who considers leadership an opportunity for service.

Author Unknown

Reprinted from the *Blueprint Prepared for Local Leaders* by the National Education Association, Revised April, 1958.

Contents

Part One. Nursing Team Leadership—A Challenge to Today's Professional Nurse

Chapter 1

WHAT IS THE PLACE OF THE PROFESSIONAL NURSE
IN NURSING TODAY? 3
    Aims of the Hospital 3
    Definitions of Nursing Care 3
    Nursing—Yesterday and Today 6
    Why Team Nursing... 10
    Study Questions 14
    Part One Bibliography 14

Part Two. You and Your Team Work Together

Chapter 2

TEAM MEMBERS ARE PEOPLE, TOO................................. 19
    People and Their Basic Needs 19
    People and Their Feelings 23
    People and Their Attitudes 24
    People Are Not All Alike 25
    Study Questions 27

Chapter 3

LEADERSHIP—WHAT IS IT?.. 28
    Some Definitions.. 28
    General Types of Leadership 29
    Leadership in Administration 30
    Leadership in Supervision..................................... 35
    Study Questions 37

Chapter 4

LEADERSHIP IN TEAM NURSING.. 38
    Your Type of Leadership—Directive or Creative?..... 38
    Techniques of Team Leadership............................. 40
    The Importance of Effective Communication........... 43
    Do You Have What It Takes To Be a Leader? 49
    Study Questions 51
    Part Two Bibliography 51

Part Three. *How To Lead Your Team*

Chapter 5

HOW TO ORGANIZE YOUR WORK 57
    How To Prepare Yourself 57
    How To Prepare Your Team 66
    How To Give a Good Patient Report 68
    How To Make a Good Assignment 71
    How To Keep Organized 78
    Questions about Work Organization 80
    Study Questions 85

Chapter 6

HOW TO SUPERVISE YOUR TEAM 86
    Supervision and the Team Leader........................... 86
    Legal Aspects of Team Leadership.......................... 87
    Supervision Is the Key to Team Leadership 90
    Supervision Uses Teaching 91
    What Areas Should Be Supervised?......................... 97
    Techniques of Observation..................................... 98
    How To Use the Information Obtained Through
        Observation 106
    Supervision and Human Relations........................... 110
    Problems That You Cannot Solve 113
    Questions Asked about Supervision 114
    Study Questions 115

Chapter 7

HOW TO CONDUCT THE TEAM CONFERENCE 117
    Purposes of the Team Conference 117
    Planning for the Conference 119
    Conducting the Conference 123
    Questions Asked about the Team Conference 129
    Study Questions 130

CONTENTS

Chapter 8

HOW TO MAKE AND TO USE NURSING CARE PLANS 132
    Purposes of the Nursing Care Plan 132
    Essential Parts of a Patient Care Plan 133
    When and How To Begin the Nursing Care Plan ... 135
    How To Plan Individual Nursing Care 136
    How To Keep Nursing Care Plans Up to Date 142
    How To Use the Nursing Care Plans 143
    Questions Asked about Nursing Care Plans 144
    Study Questions 146
    Part Three Bibliography 149

Part Four. The Team and Other Hospital Personnel

Chapter 9

TEAMWORK MUST EXTEND BEYOND THE TEAM 155
    Cooperation between the Teams 155
    The Head Nurse and Team Nursing 156
    The Nursing Student and Team Nursing 161
    The Clinical Instructor and Team Nursing 162
    The Nursing Supervisor and Team Nursing 163
    The Licensed Practical Nurse and Team Nursing...... 164
    Study Questions 166
    Part Four Bibliography 166

INDEX 169

PART ONE

Nursing Team Leadership— A Challenge to Today's Professional Nurse

*For Yesterday is but a Dream,
And To-morrow is only a Vision;
But To-day well-lived makes every
    Yesterday a Dream of Happiness
And every To-morrow a Vision of Hope.
Look well therefore to this Day!*

from The Salutation of the Dawn,
from the Sanskrit.

1

WHAT IS THE PLACE OF THE PROFESSIONAL NURSE IN NURSING TODAY?

AIMS OF THE HOSPITAL

The primary aim of any hospital is to care for the sick. Additional aims, such as research and education, are formulated only because they will eventually lead either to the prevention of disease or to the improvement of patient care.

Each department within the hospital enlarges on this primary aim by relating its specific objectives and activities to the patient and his welfare. Thus, the dietary department is concerned with the nutritional care of the patient; the housekeeping department with the care of the patient's environment; the laboratory and x-ray departments with diagnostic and therapeutic techniques designed to help the patient in his recovery; and so on throughout every division within the hospital. In the nursing service department the aim becomes that of giving continuous good nursing care to each patient.

DEFINITIONS OF NURSING CARE

During the last ten years some phrases have been coined to

describe various kinds of patient care. Perhaps it would be helpful to consider these terms in an attempt to determine if they can be used interchangeably or if each has a different meaning.

Total Patient Care. The first of these phases is *total patient care or comprehensive nursing care.* What is the meaning of this phrase? It is usually defined as meeting all the needs of the patient—emotional, spiritual, physical, environmental, social, economic, and rehabilitative, and includes all teaching needed in any of these areas. Total care recognizes the patient as a member of his family and his community and strives to help the patient and the family to make the necessary adjustments to his limitations. The nurse recognizes that many people will contribute to the total care of her patient and that she will need to act as guide, teacher, and coordinator to some who render service to her patient.

The professional nurse knows that the patient with heart failure needs rest—physical and mental. His drugs, treatments, food, and nursing care, as well as his environment and rehabilitation, must be planned with this need in mind. He must be taught which activities, foods, and drugs are good for him and why. He must also learn which ones are contraindicated so that he will understand and derive the most benefit from his hospital care. He must realize the effect that emotions may have on his condition, and he must be helped to understand what to do about his job, and his place in his family and community. This is total patient care.

Individualized Patient Care. What then of the phrase—*individualized patient care* or, as it is sometimes called, *patient-centered care?* Is it the same as total care? The answer is yes except that it goes a step further. This phrase implies the application of total care on a more personal level. Perhaps an illustration will clarify this. During a clinical discussion about the care of a patient with compensated heart disease who was almost ready to go home, the instructor and a group of nursing students were talking about what this patient needed to be taught in order to care for himself at home. Glibly the students listed such items as low-salt diet, rest, and some of the activities he should avoid. The instructor, probing for a show of more understanding of the patient as an individual, asked about his home problems, what foods he liked or disliked, what specific activities were a necessary part of his home life, and, if contraindicated by his heart condition, what modifications could be suggested. The students insisted that the patient needed to be taught that he should not walk up and down stairs at home. Finally the instructor asked if the man lived in a house where it was necessary for him to use a stairway. They did not know. This illustration demonstrates the difference between total care and individualized care.

Total care includes all the areas and all the principles that the nurse must keep in mind when caring for *any* patient with a certain condition; in individualized care, the nurse becomes acquainted with her patient as a person and seeks to understand his problems. She then refers to the principles that are defined in total care and uses those that apply to this particular patient as she plans for his care and teaching.

Total care says to promote mental rest for the patient with heart disease by explaining procedures, by giving reassurance, and by relieving his mind of worries. It does not, however, tell the nurse how to give the explanation or reassurance needed by this patient, nor does it indicate what may be worrying him or what to do to relieve those worries. The nurse who gives patient-centered care must discover these things for herself. She will soon realize that the answers to the problems of Mr. Jones cannot be used for Mr. Smith even though he may be suffering from the same condition. The guiding principles remain the same, but their application will differ because Mr. Smith and Mr. Jones are two different individuals with different problems and different responses to their environment.

Good Nursing Care. Another phrase which has different meanings to different people is *nursing care*. To some, nursing care still means the performance of procedures according to predetermined steps or established hospital policies. Frances Reiter Kreuter in her discussion of nursing care* insists that the administration of medicines, tests, and treatments is a nursing *operation* which cannot be called nursing *care* unless the nurse helps the patient during the experience. In other words, nursing responsibilities and duties are not the same as nursing care. Nurses have many duties delegated to them by the medical profession and by the hospital administration, but determining the nursing care that a patient needs and how to give it are functions belonging to the nurse alone.

Some authorities speak of nursing care as maintaining the equilibrium of the patient, doing for the patient that which he is unable to do for himself, or giving support to the patient. We hear about nursing practice, nursing techniques, nursing problems, meeting patient needs, nurse-patient relationships. Most of these are abstract terms for which nurses are still seeking concrete definitions. It is time for nurses to stop talking about what is good nursing care and formulate a specific and workable definition that can be used as a guide in the planning, giving, and evaluating of nursing care.

In the meantime, each nurse must formulate her own definition

---

*Kreuter, Frances Reiter: *What Is Good Nursing Care?* Nurs. Outlook, May, 1957, pp. 302–304.

of nursing care and establish her own goals and standards in giving that care. The work of the team will reflect the philosophy and goals of the team leader, the professional nurse.

NURSING — YESTERDAY AND TODAY

Changes in the Field of Medicine. The discovery of the principles of the microscope, the x-ray, photography, plastics, and the inventions of the twentieth century, such as the radio and television, and the use of atomic energy have added impetus to medical research. These have brought about a rapid increase in the knowledge concerning the cause and treatment of many diseases.

New drugs are being used in the treatment of measles, smallpox, herpes simplex, and influenza. Laser energy is being tried in the treatment of detached retina and certain malignant tumors. Scientists are giving the medical world additional information about the causes and treatment of certain heart, blood, and vascular diseases. The role of DNA in heredity is being studied. New and improved surgical techniques and instruments make possible, and even routine, some operations which a few years ago were unheard of. Hyperbaric surgery reduces mortality in operations on infants with congenital heart diseases. The use of intense cold in the treatment of certain conditions is being tried. Artificial hearts and lungs serve as temporary substitutes for those vital organs, and actual transplantation of organs such as kidneys, lungs, livers, spleens, and even hearts is being tried experimentally. Electronic pacemakers keep damaged hearts beating rhythmically. In several instances severed limbs have been reattached successfully. Plastic materials and certain metals are being used to replace diseased sections of the body. Many facets of psychiatry, geriatrics, public health and sanitation are receiving attention of specialists in these fields.

Although great advances have been made, much remains to be done. Increasing longevity of life is creating problems in health as well as in social and economic areas. Cancer and the common cold remain unconquered. The incidence of veneral diseases has increased. Epidemics of encephalitis, infectious hepatitis, and drug-resistant meningitis also point up the fact that we have not yet controlled communicable diseases. Continued advancement in space exploration necessitates research in space medicine.

The family doctor of yesteryear is almost unknown today. The quantity and complexity of medical knowledge have resulted in specialization and the increased use of consultation. Technicians, under the supervision of physicians who direct their work, are using the intricate equipment found in many areas of the modern hospital, for example, in the laboratory, the x-ray and the physical therapy departments.

Changes in Hospitals. Hospitals have also changed. At the beginning of the century a hospital was a big dismal building, thought by many people to be a place of death. Now architecture and interior decoration are changing the physical appearance of the hospital while progress in medical science continues to eliminate the dangers that previously lurked within its walls. Gone are the high somber tan or dingy white walls and the narrow bare windows. The effect of color on the emotional response of the individual, and hence on his recovery, is now recognized; consequently, every effort is made to make the hospital bright and attractive as well as efficient and safe. Nursing stations are now being planned so that the nurse can observe quickly and communicate easily with each patient.

Automation is becoming a part of hospital life. Intricate machines monitor the vital signs of patients, keeping minute by minute records of their progress. Data processing machines are used to maintain patient records, to plan staffing, and in other ways to relieve people of the quantity of paper work. These machines, in turn, have made necessary new knowledge and skills. The use of disposable materials, including premixed infant formulas, medications, and equipment such as needles, syringes, and linen supplies, just to name a few, decreases the time needed to prepare and maintain these supplies as well as lessens the chance of infection.

In order to make more efficient use of personnel and equipment, some hospitals are grouping patients according to the care that they need. This system of progressive patient care includes an intensive care unit for the critically ill, a recovery room for patients immediately following surgery, regular care for the average patient, and minimal care or self-care units for convalescent patients and others who are ambulatory.

Changes in Social and Economic Conditions. With the decline in death rates has come a rise in the average age of the total population. A rise in the birth rate, combined with a drop in infant mortality, is causing a condition which statisticians and sociologists are calling the "population explosion." This means that more and more people will need the services of doctors, nurses, and hospitals.

In addition to the increase in the number of people, several other factors are influencing the trend toward the greater use of medical and hospital facilities. The family is no longer a closely knit, stable, more or less independent entity. The shift is now away from the care of infirm, aged and ill persons by their own families. More and more the care of these individuals is assumed by service organizations such as nursing homes and hospitals. The increased amount of information about health and disease, now being given in school and in popular literature, has made most people more health conscious. Along with this increased interest in health has come an increase in the number of subscriptions to the various hospitalization and health plans, thus making medical care more readily available to the public even though hospital rates have increased. Doctors can no longer meet the demand for their services on a home-call basis, nor do they have available in their offices all the equipment and other facilities necessary for diagnostic and therapeutic care of their patients; therefore, they prescribe hospitalization.

Changes in Nursing and Nursing Education. In the past nurses did many of the housekeeping tasks around the hospital or home in addition to attending to the wants of their patients. Their duties were simple and entailed little knowledge or understanding of the patient's disease or the doctor's treatment. The nurse simply did as she was told. However, to keep pace with the changes in medicine, nurses have found it necessary to assume increasingly complex duties, to learn to work with new equipment safely and effectively and, consequently, to acquire more knowledge and understanding of medical diagnosis and treatment and of nursing itself. Various techniques, such as the administration of intravenous fluids, once thought to be within the realm of doctors only, are now being delegated to the professional nurse. As the care of the patient moved out of the home and into the hospital, the nursing profession found that it must supply more and more of that personal element hitherto provided by the patient's family. As a result of these changes, nurses and their professional organizations are trying to evaluate, define, and set up standards of nursing care.

The increase in the size and numbers of hospitals, the increased daily census of patients, the shortening of the work week, and the growing number of complex skills and responsibilities have increased the demand for nurses beyond the available supply. New fields of endeavor, continually opening up to nurses in industry and public health, are taking some nurses who otherwise might be available for service in hospitals. An apparent decrease in the number of available professional nurses to care for patients has caused an increase in the use of practical nurses and ancillary personnel.

Nursing education is confronted with the task of preparing the nurse to assume her role in society and in nursing. But what is that role? Several basic nursing programs are in existence — each with the expressed or implied objective of preparing nurses for first level positions, in other words, as a staff nurse who gives bedside care to patients. But does the phrase, "first level," imply

WHAT IS THE PLACE OF THE PROFESSIONAL NURSE IN NURSING TODAY?   9

the existence of other levels above this? Bedside nursing has assumed the lowest status value in nursing, usually assigned to practical nurses or aides. Yet what is the role of the professional nurse if not to give nursing care?

Marguerite Kakosh* says:

> "Bedside care seems so much less important than the work of the head nurse or supervisor. 'I'm just a staff nurse' is the common remark. 'Today I was an aide. I did all the work that an aide does—gave baths, dressed and fed patients, assisted them into wheelchairs.' Was there really any difference in the practice of the aide and the nurse? Perhaps there is little reason to value it any more highly. Until we are *able* and *enabled* to practice that quality of care that has inherent in it a growing source of satisfaction, we cannot expect respect for it. . . .
>
> "Do we know *what* we are educating nurses for? Is my care the same as that given by the auxiliary? If there is no difference, then the *profession* of nursing will die and only the *occupation* of nursing will continue to exist!"

Members of the various health groups see the nurse in widely differing roles. Making a diagnosis and prescribing the treatment of the illness of a patient is the primary responsibility of the physician. Traditionally, the nurse has been considered one who "waits on" the doctor and performs the therapeutic techniques that he prescribes. On the other hand, hospital administrators think of the nurse as one who is capable of managing a section of the hospital, carrying out all administrative policies of the institution. In addition, the number of allied therapy personnel—laboratory and x-ray technicians, physical and occupational therapists, inhalation therapists, intravenous therapy teams, etc.—is increasing daily. The nurse is often responsible for coordinating the services of these people into the patient's schedule of care. As a result, she cannot find time to give nursing care to the patient. In other words, the nurse has allowed herself to become an assistant doctor, an assistant hospital administrator, a traffic manager, a service coordinator—a jack-of-all-trades but master of none. Although these duties are important to the patient's welfare, they do not constitute the giving of nursing care, which is the nurse's primary function. In her concern to perform these secondary duties, the nurse tends to neglect her main responsibility to the patient. In fact, she often delegates much of his care to ancillary workers.

In her primary role the professional nurse must be allowed to operate independently yet cooperatively with all members of the health team. As a specialist in nursing she assesses the patient's needs, looks for nursing problems, determines what nursing care is needed and how it should be given. In other words, she makes a "nursing diagnosis" and prescribes the nursing care needed to

---

*Kakosh, Marguerite: *Shortages: Nurses or Nursing?* Reprinted by permission from the *Canad. Nurse*, 60:2:131, 1960.

help the patient to attain and to maintain a state of balance during this time of stress.

The necessity for greater understanding of the patient and the tensions imposed upon him by his illness along with the changes in nursing philosophy and responsibilities of the professional nurse suggest the need for specialization in nursing. There is much talk about "freeing the nurse to nurse." Ward managers may take over the administrative and coordinative duties of the head nurse, leaving her time for her real nursing function, planning and evaluating the nursing care for each patient and supervising her staff who give that care. The present trend of thought also suggests the need for two categories of registered nurses, each a specialist in her own area. One would be the *nurse clinician* who, because of her greater knowledge of physiological and behavioral sciences, is a specialist in determining how to help the patient most effectively. She would be directly involved in patient care and would help other nurses and ancillary workers to find solutions to nursing problems. The other specialist would be the *nurse technician* who acquires greater understanding and skill in the actual performance of nursing techniques and delegated medical therapy. These two persons would work with other nursing personnel in providing the care that each patient needs.

In order to prepare nurses to function in their primary role, nursing education insists that the educational program should emphasize knowledge of the physiological, behavioral, and social sciences as a foundation to understanding the patient as an individual and administering safe, effective nursing care. The trend is away from the apprenticeship training which emphasized those skills which were necessary in giving physical care to patients.

WHY TEAM NURSING

Problems Confronting Nursing Today. Nursing is in a state of evolution. The pressure of striving for recognition as a profession, combined with the changes in duties, responsibilities, and changes in the attitudes of nurses themselves, have caused conflicts between nurses and auxiliary workers and a sense of frustration within the nurses themselves. Tradition has defined the practice of nursing as the direct personal care of the sick. In present-day practice, the nurse finds herself concerned more and more with technical, supervisory, and administrative duties, and is less and less able to be at the bedside of her patients. This conflict between what the professional nurse has been taught nursing to be and what she now finds herself doing is the major problem confronting nursing today.

Because confusion exists concerning what nursing is and what nurses should do, discrepancies sometimes occur between what the nursing student is taught and what she is expected to do when she graduates. As a student she is taught patient-centered care. Yet when she leaves the shelter of the nursing program, she may find that her work tends to become "procedure-centered" or "task-oriented" rather than "patient-centered." In small hospitals, especially, the young graduate may find that she is expected to "take charge" of a nursing station because she is the only registered nurse available. Usually her education for a "first level" position has given her very little instruction or experience in administrative or supervisory activities.

Because nurses themselves are not sure what their responsibilities *do* include, they judge their work on the basis of techniques alone, rather than on what their care could mean to the patient. In view of some of the criticism of hospitals and nurses, it appears that the nursing profession is failing to give what the public considers to be good nursing care. Studies seem to indicate that a patient is most concerned with his physical comfort, with being told what to expect, and with having his questions answered. In other words, nurses were most often criticized for their lack of communication and consideration of the personal needs of the patient. On the other hand, these same studies indicated that nurses felt that giving treatments and medications on time, and maintaining a safe environment were the most important aspects of the patient's care.

Nurses apparently are failing to understand their patients and, consequently, are unable to make the patients understand them. The professional nurse of today believes that, due to the pressure of doing so many things for the patient, she is wasting time if she spends a few minutes "just talking" with the patient. Nevertheless, communication is one of the most important phases of nursing care, for in no other way can the patient be helped to understand his treatment, his progress, or to solve his problems. It is impossible, for example, to administer a pill that will allow the patient to understand why he is afraid or to realize the relationship between his fears and some of his physical symptoms.

In the light of the previous definitions of patient care, are we being fair to the nurses' aide, with her three to four weeks of on-the-job training, if we expect her to do more than follow procedures as taught? Usually she has no knowledge, or at best a limited amount, about the patient's disease and its effect on his physical, emotional, and environmental needs. Nevertheless, she is the one who spends many hours at the patient's bedside, talking with him as she works, and answering his questions. How can we be sure that the information or the nursing care so given is correct and best for the patient? The aim of her training is implied in her title—nurses' aide, one who works under the direction of a professional nurse.

Even the licensed practical nurse with her 1 year education has, for the most part, only technical training in the performance of relatively simple procedures. Although she receives a greater amount of information concerning disease conditions, she does not learn about the emotional, or even all the physical reactions of the patients. Again are we being fair to expect her to give individualized care to all patients? The stated aim of the schools of practical nursing is to train a person to work directly under the direction of a doctor or a professional nurse.

Traditionally, the head nurse has been the person who is responsible for the direction and supervision of her staff, each person being directly responsible to her. Today, in view of present conditions in many hospitals, the head nurse has no time to give more than cursory direction, help, and supervision. Under the functional method of assignment, staff nurses have only occasional personal contact with the ancillary workers, and frequently their only contact with the patients comes during the administration of medications or treatments. They do not have the authority, or the opportunity, to direct and supervise the care being given by other personnel. There is little communication among the personnel themselves, and little or no coordination between the fragments of nursing care that each person is assigned to give. The nurses' aide and practical nurse who spend the most time with the patient, talking with him, and becoming acquainted with his personal problems, are unable to make use of this information to help the patient understand his condition or to solve his problems. Nevertheless, according to Frances Kreuter, unless the patient has been so helped, nursing care has not been given.

Team Nursing Will Help Solve Some of These Problems. Team nursing was never devised to make up for an inadequate staff; however, it was devised to provide better nursing care with the available staff. The team, by working closely together, can give better care because the abilities of each team member are utilized, and all nursing care is closely guided and supervised by a professional nurse who is the team leader. Patient-centered care is implemented by the daily team conference when the entire team discusses the needs of each patient and devises ways of meeting those needs. A written nursing care plan, which is to be used by every team member, is then made and is revised as the patient's condition changes. The team leader decides what person on her team is best qualified to care for each patient. In this way the professional nurse helps all members of her team learn what is best for each patient and insures good nursing care with individual consideration for the patient's needs and problems, although she may not be the one who actually gives the care or answers the patient's questions.

Not only are there insufficient professional nurses to give bedside care, but there are also too few nurses trained in administration and supervision to fill the available positions. Some schools of nursing include one or two courses designed to help the nursing student acquire a basic knowledge of the principles of administration. Very few schools, however, offer the student a well-planned experience in learning how to apply these principles in an acutal situation. Yet in many hospitals a recent graduate, or even a senior nursing student, is expected to "take charge" with little or no help from a more experienced person.

In team nursing the professional nurse, as team leader, can gain practical experience in democratic leadership by directing and supervising her team. She can learn how to work effectively with many kinds of people; how to establish and maintain good human relations; how to plan, direct, supervise, and evaluate the work of others; and how to coordinate the activities of a number of people working together. In other words, team leadership is a practical means of preparing every nurse to learn some administrative duties and to become more skilled in giving nursing care.

The Challenge of Team Leadership. Every nurse, if she believes that she belongs to a profession, must be a leader. People look to her for help and guidance, especially in those areas pertaining to health. She must have a genuine liking for people and be sincerely interested in their welfare. As a professional person she must also be active in community affairs.

Leadership in team nursing offers a special challenge to the graduate nurse for making use of all the knowledge, understanding, and skills that her training has provided. She must be able to plan, give, supervise, and evaluate nursing care; to coordinate hospital and community resources for the benefit of each patient; to make decisions wisely and calmly as the need arises; to work harmoniously and communicate effectively with all kinds of people; to seek constantly to improve in the practice of her profession; and to set an example not only as a good nurse but also as a good citizen.

Every team leader, if her leadership is to be effective, must know the basic principles of administration, supervision, guidance, and teaching and be able to apply them as she works with her team. Sometimes it is easier to know *what* to do than it is to determine *how* to do it. It is the aim of this book to give the basic principles which every person needs to know for effective leadership and to show their practical application in situations that are commonly found in team nursing.

STUDY QUESTIONS

1. What do you think is the main contribution of the nurse to the doctor-nurse-patient relationship? Why?
2. What do you think is the most important contribution the nurse can make to the patient? Why?
3. How would you answer when someone says, "I didn't see a nurse during the entire week I was in the hospital"?
4. What do *you* mean when you say someone is a *good* patient? Analyze your meaning.
5. What do you mean when you describe someone as being a *good* nurse?
6. What is the difference between the function of the health team and the function of the nursing team?
7. List as many changes as you can that have occurred in the field of medicine in your own hospital in the last five years. What brought about each change? What were the effects of each change on the duties and responsibilities of the professional nurse?
8. Formulate your own definition of nursing care.
9. Select one nursing technique and set up a guide to evaluate the nursing care given during the performance of that technique. Analyze the criteria you have set up. How many of these are based solely on performance of steps of a procedure or established hospital policy? Will your guide help you to evaluate nursing care according to your definition in question 8?
10. Observe a registered nurse other than a head nurse or supervisor. List everything that she does. Classify each as to whether it is delegated medical therapy, related hospital administration, correlating services of allied health groups, or giving direct nursing care, etc. Compare the results of your observation according to number of activities and time spent on each.

PART ONE BIBLIOGRAPHY

Angrist, Shirley: *Nursing Care: The Dream and the Reality.* Am. J. Nursing, 65:4:66, April, 1965.

Barclay, Goldie N.: *Keeping Trained Personnel at the Bedside.* Hospitals, 37:2:64, Jan. 16, 1964.

Bean, Margaret, et al.: *Monitoring Through Electronics.* Am. J. Nursing, 63:4:65, April, 1963.

Bixler, Genevieve K., and Bixler, Roy W.: *The Professional Status of Nursing.* Am. J. Nursing, 59:8:1142, Aug., 1959.

Brackett, Mary E., and Fogt, Joan R.: *Is Comprehensive Nursing Care a Realistic Goal?* Nurs. Outlook, 9:7:402, July, 1961.

Bratton, Jimmie K.: *A Definition of Comprehensive Nursing Care.* Nurs. Outlook, 9:8:481, Aug., 1961.

Cherescavish, Gertrude: *The Expanding Role of the Professional Nurse in a Hospital.* Nursing Forum, 3:4:9, 1964.

Coladarci, Arthur P.: *What About that Word Profession.* Am. J. Nursing, 63:10:116; Oct., 1963.

Defining Nursing by Doing Nursing. (Editorial) Am. J. Nursing, 61:12:49, Dec., 1961.

Editorial, Nursing Science, F. A. Davis Company, Philadelphia. April, 1963, page 41.

Freeing the Nurse to Nurse. (Editorial) Am. J. Nursing, 64:3:72, March, 1964.

Fritz, Edna L.: *Philosophy, A Means of Shaping Reality.* Minnesota League for Nursing. Bulletin, 12:3:3, Feb., 1964.

From Blinking to Thinking. (Editorial) Am. J. Nursing, 61:11:55, Nov., 1961.

WHAT IS THE PLACE OF THE PROFESSIONAL NURSE IN NURSING TODAY?

Hall, Lydia E.: *Nursing—What Is It?* Canadian Nurse, 60:2:150, Feb., 1964.
Hamilton, T. Stewart: *Changing Patterns in Medical and Hospital Administration.* Hospitals, 37:11:31, June 1, 1963.
Hassenplug, Lulu Wolf: *The World of Nursing—2000 A.D.* Am. J. Nursing, 62:8:100, Aug., 1962.
Henderson, Virginia: *The Nature of Nursing.* Am. J. Nursing, 64:8:62, Aug., 1964.
Jahoda, Marie: *Nursing as A Profession.* Am. J. Nursing, 61:7:52, July, 1961.
Johnson, Dorothy E.: *A Philosophy of Nursing.* Nurs. Outlook, 7:4:198, April, 1959.
Johnson, Dorothy E.: *Consequences for Patients and Personnel.* Am. J. Nursing, 62:5:96, May, 1962.
Johnson, Dorothy E.: *Patterns in Professional Nursing Education.* Nurs. Outlook, 9:10:608, Oct., 1961.
Johnson, Dorothy E.: *Significance of Nursing Care.* Am. J. Nursing, 61:11:63, Nov., 1961.
Kakosh, Marguerite: *Shortages: Nurses or Nursing?* Canadian Nurse, 60:2:131, Feb., 1960.
Kreuter, Frances R.: *What Is Good Nursing Care?* Nurs. Outlook, 5:5:302, May, 1957.
Kurtz, Richard A., and Flaming, Karl H.: *Professionalism—The Case of Nurses.* Am. J. Nursing, 63:1:75, Jan., 1963.
Lambertsen, Eleanor: *If Nursing Has Changed, so Have Doctors and Hospitals.* Modern Hospital, 99:5:124, Nov., 1962.
Lindsey, Margaret: *Professional Standards—Whose Responsibility?* Am. J. Nursing, 62:11:84, Nov., 1962.
Marie, Sister Charles: *Nursing Needs More Freedom.* Am. J. Nursing, 62:7:53, July, 1962.
Marie, Sister Charles: *Tomorrow's Reality.* Nursing Science, F. A. Davis Company, Philadelphia. Dec. 1963, page 332.
Mercadante, Lucille R.: *Unit Manager Plan Gives Nurses More Time to Care for the Patients.* Modern Hospital, 99:2:73, Aug., 1962.
Montag, Mildred L.: *Technical Education in Nursing?* Am. J. Nursing, 63:5:101, May, 1963.
Mullane, Mary Kelly: *Care Systems and Nursing Education.* Nurs. Outlook, 11:10:740, Oct., 1963.
Mullane, Mary K.: *Nursing Service and Patient Care.* Hospital Progress, 44:11:85, Nov., 1963.
Nahm, Helen: *Nursing Dimensions and Realities.* Am. J. Nursing, 65:6:96, June, 1965.
New, Peter Kong-Ming: *Another Approach to Professionalism.* Am. J. Nursing, 65:2:124, Feb., 1965.
Newton, Mildred E.: *What's Ahead for Nursing and NLN?* Nurs. Outlook, 9:10:600, Oct., 1961.
Perkins, Erline W.: *The Registered Nurse—a Professional Person.* 63:2:90, Feb., 1963.
Porter, Elizabeth K.: *Traditions and Realities.* Am. J. Nursing, 63:11:M3, Nov., 1963.
Perspectives for Nursing. National League for Nursing. No. 11-1166, 1965.
Rogers, Martha E.: *Some Comments on the Theoretical Basis of Nursing Practice.* Nursing Science, F. A. Davis Company, Philadelphia, April, 1963, page 11.
Schlotfeldt, Rozella: *Responsible Leadership: Whom for What?* Nursing Science, F. A. Davis Company, Philadelphia, Dec., 1963, page 341.
Scott, Jessie M.: *Seeing Nursing Activities as They Are.* Am. J. Nursing, 62:11:70, Nov., 1962.
Smith, Dorothy M.: *Myth and Method in Nursing Practice.* Am. J. Nursing, 64:2:68, Feb., 1964.
Stevenson, Neva M.: *The Better Utilization of Licensed Practical Nurses.* Nurs. Outlook, 13:7:340, July, 1965.
Taylor, Carol: *How Unit Managers Work for Us.* The Modern Hospital, 99:2:69, Aug., 1962.
Walker, Virginia, and Hawkins, James L.: *Management: A Factor in Clinical Nursing.* Nurs. Outlook, 13:2:57, Feb., 1965.

Wheeler, Dorothy V.: *Who Determines Nursing's Destiny?* Am. J. Nursing, 63:12:65, Dec., 1963.

Whitaker, Judith G.: *The Changing Role of the Professional Nurse in the Hospital.* Am. J. Nursing, 62:2:65, Feb., 1962.

White, Dorothy T.: *Have Our Values in Nursing Really Changed—or Were We Sidetracked?* Nursing Science, F. A. Davis Company, Philadelphia, April, 1963, page 48.

Wiedenbach, Ernestine: *The Helping Art of Nursing.* Am. J. Nursing, 63:11:54, Nov., 1963.

_____ PART TWO

You and Your Team Work Together

We are here not to get all we can out of life for ourselves, but to try to make the lives of others happier.

from Life of Sir William Osler,
by Harvey Cushing.
Vol. I Chapter 22.

2

TEAM MEMBERS ARE PEOPLE, TOO

Because of our concern for the patient, his needs and his problems, we sometimes forget that the members of our team are human beings, not unfeeling robots, and that all of us have needs that must be satisfied. We can understand the problems and emotions of our patients only to the degree that we understand ourselves and the vital part that the satisfaction of our basic needs plays in the development of each one of us as individuals.

PEOPLE AND THEIR BASIC NEEDS

The Need for Recognition. Every person wants to be recognized as an individual, a person with certain abilities as well as with certain limitations. Everyone wants to feel that he or she is important to someone else. Normally, this need for recognition results in certain forms of behavior. For example, creativeness, possessiveness, mastery, rivalry, and display stem from the fact that the human being is motivated to project his ego upon his immediate surroundings.

This desire to be somebody is healthy as long as it remains within normal limits, but if it becomes exaggerated, the individual becomes overly concerned with self and less concerned with others. He becomes selfish, boastful, overcritical, and forgetful of the feelings of others. He seeks in every possible way to draw attention to himself. The words *I, me,* and *mine* play a very important part in his conversation as well as in his thinking.

As a team leader you can use to advantage this need for personal recognition by giving praise and showing appreciation whenever they are deserved. Sincere praise makes the person feel worthwhile and important, stimulating her to continue her good work. Praise is like salt—a little, wisely used, brings out the good qualities; too much spoils them. Sometimes all that is necessary is a simple "thank you," spoken directly to a member of your team, showing that you recognize her intentions and are grateful for her help.

On the other hand, you will need to control the individual who shows signs of wanting too much attention. The desire for recognition is related to, and dependent upon, other needs. It is possible that one or more of these are not being met to her satisfaction although her behavior seems to point to one area only. Study the individual carefully. Analyze her responses in various situations in an effort to determine their cause. Show appreciation for her satisfactory behavior and, whenever possible, ignore that which is less commendable, thus indirectly helping her to behave in a more acceptable manner.

As team leader it is important that you control your own desire to feel important, lest it overshadow the consideration you should give to your team members and thus destroy your effectiveness as a leader.

Nursing students and staff nurses alike complain, "No one pays any attention to us when we do things right, only when we do something wrong." In many cases their complaint is justified because someone forgot their need for recognition and a feeling of self-worth.

The Need To Belong. Every individual desires to be part of a group. This goes beyond merely wanting to be with people. We are all naturally gregarious, but if the need to belong is to be satisfied, we must feel that we are accepted by others and that they like us. The individual wishes to feel accepted by the entire group because, through this affiliation, he gains the prestige that is accorded to the group as a whole.

This desire to belong is demonstrated most vividly by the teenager and his gang or her crowd. As evidence of belonging, everyone must dress alike, speak alike, have the same mannerisms. We find this group-consciousness just as strong among those adults who join lodges and clubs of all kinds.

In a hospital or nursing home many individuals share in caring for the patient—some directly, some indirectly—but each one is very important to the welfare of each patient. How many of us would be able to, or would care to, go to the engine room and maintain the equipment there so that our patients would have light, heat, and hot water? How many of us would care to wash and iron all the linen for our patients, or to prepare all their food, or do

TEAM MEMBERS ARE PEOPLE, TOO

all the cleaning? There was a time when this work was considered a normal part of the nurse's duties. But not any more. Now many persons work together to provide for the comfort and well-being of the patient, and no single worker is more important than another.

In the hospital, uniforms often designate the status of the worker. Thus, we have dietary workers wearing one color, housekeeping workers wearing another, and nursing students still another—each color a badge of belonging to a particular group. Sometimes this organization takes on all the aspects of a caste system in which each individual associates with or feels at ease with only the other members of her own work-group. Usually, in this kind of atmosphere, there is very little mutual understanding or rapport among the various groups.

In team nursing each person on the team is concerned with giving nursing care to a patient; yet each person is important to the total functioning of the team in direct proportion to the utilization of her skills and abilities.

As team leader you should encourage the development of team spirit by emphasizing *our* instead of *my* and *your,* and by making each one feel that her contribution is important to the entire group. Only through your help, encouragement, and example will each person become an active participant in the work of the team.

Occasionally, you may find a person who does not seem to feel this need to belong. She appears to prefer to work and be alone. She does not readily enter into group conversations. She may even act disdainful of the others, giving the impression that she thinks she is better than they. This behavior may be only a defense. Actually, she may want to be a member of the group, but because she is afraid that they do not want her, she hides behind her seeming wish to be left alone. You will need to encourage and provide opportunities for her to participate in group activities. In addition, you should suggest that the rest of the team include her in their conversations, and that they ask for her help, offering to help her in return.

The Need for Understanding. Everyone wants to express herself so that others will understand her and her problems, limitations, fears, hopes, and desires. The need to understand others is just as great. Each person wants to know what others expect of her, what her responsibilities are, and how well she is meeting those responsibilities.

This need for understanding is closely related to the need for recognition since both are based on respect and admiration. We want to be looked up to; yet it is just as important that we ourselves have someone to whom we can look for help and understanding.

Problems are bound to arise if this need is ignored. If one

believes that it is unnecessary to understand others, she is likely to become cold, aloof, and uninterested in others and their problems. On the other hand, when there is no desire to be understood, one may become uncommunicative, displaying very little emotion, apparently caring little about the reactions of others toward herself.

If this need to understand and be understood is exaggerated, the person may become so anxious to gain respect that she will seek to obtain it by any means. She may become demanding, expect to have her opinion consulted often, and be excessively anxious to please for fear others will not respect her. She may spend much time discussing the problems of others, give praise lavishly, or become too lenient and overly tolerant of their work and actions in the hope that this will make them like her more.

As team leader you have an important part in satisfying the needs of each of your team members. Yet your ability to satisfy them is dependent upon your own ability to understand and to be understood. If you feel sorry for yourself, believing that no one understands you and your problems, your loneliness and resentment will be passed on to your team. They, in turn, will feel that you do not understand them or their problems. You must take an individual interest in each person, seeking to learn the meaning of what they leave unsaid as well as of what they say. Help them to know exactly what they are to do, then let them know how well they are meeting your expectations. If they are not measuring up, determine why; perhaps a need for better understanding exists.

The Need for Stimulation and Personal Growth. Change is stimulating. Change may also be a means of providing a person with the opportunity, as well as the incentive, to acquire new knowledge and understanding, to think new thoughts, to solve more difficult problems, or to learn new skills. Without this stimulation comes boredom, and with boredom comes lack of interest in doing a good job.

The amount of stimulation needed by each individual will vary from person to person, but usually the desire to have some new experiences is always present. Some people will try constantly to see and do new things and will become unhappy when forced to perform "routine" tasks day after day. Other individuals feel more content when their duties entail the performance of the same activities over and over. Such a person may have either a limited intelligence or feelings of inferiority and insecurity. In either case, she is very likely to become upset and unhappy when confronted with new situations.

Providing opportunities to satisfy the desire for personal growth in the various members of your team is one of the challenging aspects of team leadership. You must plan carefully and give close supervision to those individuals who, in their eagerness for new experiences, may thoughtlessly engage in activities that, for the safety of the patient, they should not do. You will need to use all your powers of persuasion to help such persons understand the importance of "routine" tasks in relation to total patient care and will need to show them ways of increasing their experience and skill while performing these duties. Nursing students (and some graduate nurses too) sometimes become bored with giving baths because they feel that other aspects of patient care are so much more exciting and important. They need your help to understand that the importance is not in the giving of the bath itself but in providing a time for the patient to talk out his problems with someone who is capable of helping him.

You must encourage the person who needs new experiences in order to increase her learning and skills. Provide her with the opportunity to perform a single new activity along with her usual work. Give her the necessary help and moral support for performing this task; make the experience a satisfying one by assuring a successful performance through proper preparation and supervision. Do not forget to praise her when she is finished. Soon you will find that you have a dependable team member who can assume much more responsibility.

Occasionally, you may find that you must work with a person who is intellectually incapable of performing more than routine tasks. In this case, you should organize your work in such a way that you make full use of this person's abilities, thereby giving others more time to perform the more complex duties.

The Need for Security. Everyone must be able to depend upon something or someone, to predict with reasonable accuracy what will happen to her, and to know how others feel toward her. In other words, she must have that comfortable feeling of security if she is to function to her fullest capacity. This feeling of security is the end result of meeting and satisfying the need for recognition, for belonging, for understanding, and for new experiences. The person who feels secure can meet the problems of life with equanimity and can work out acceptable solutions to these problems with a minimum amount of frustration.

PEOPLE AND THEIR FEELINGS

Feelings may be pleasant or unpleasant and are the result of a person's response either to his environment or to something that happens with herself. Feelings so intense that they affect the internal organs, resulting not only in a mental reaction but in a physical one as well, are called emotions.

When a person's basic needs are satisfied, there is a feeling of pleasure, happiness, and enthusiasm. The person is at peace with herself and with the world. Minor annoyances fail to disturb her since she is able either to shrug them off or to face and overcome them.

If a person's needs are ignored or are not met to her satisfaction, she experiences an unpleasant feeling, which may become so intense that it becomes an emotion, such as anger, jealousy, hate, fear, or discouragement. When this occurs, her response to her immediate surroundings is also affected. Often she will vent her emotions upon someone who had nothing to do with starting this chain reaction. For example, a nurse, when reprimanded by a doctor because a patient did not receive a treatment as directed, was unable to assert herself with the doctor. Instead, she vented her feelings of frustration and anger upon another member of the staff, thereby restoring somewhat her feeling of self-worth.

As team leader you must keep in mind that your own emotional responses, along with those of your team members, will have a profound effect upon team spirit and upon the quality of nursing care that they give. You must try to provide situations that will give your team a feeling of pleasure. You should also try either to minimize those situations that will result in feelings of frustration or other unpleasant emotions, or to help the person understand and control her reactions to the situation.

PEOPLE AND THEIR ATTITUDES

Many of your reactions are the result of, either consciously or unconsciously, learned behavior. These reactions are called attitudes. You do not usually develop them in response to rational or critical thinking based on fact, but rather acquire them through your past experiences in your social environment. You have acquired attitudes toward many things—food, religion, politics, strikes, nationalities, war, team nursing, supervisors, office workers, janitors, farmers, practical nurses, etc. Have your beliefs come about because you collected all available facts, did your own critical thinking, then decided what you wanted to believe about each other?

One instructor in Fundamentals of Nursing had her freshman students fill out a questionnaire at the end of their first six months. These students had almost completed their classroom instruction in basic nursing procedures and had had some experience in caring for patients. Some of the answers showed that, in spite of classroom instruction related to attitudes toward patients, students seemed to retain many of the attitudes that they had had before entering nursing. One question asked what effect the education, age, place in the family, or wealth of a patient would have on the nursing care that the student would give. Following are some of the answers:

> "A person who has no schooling is a moron."
> "People who are educated are easier to get along with."
> "Old people are inclined to be bossy."
> "The youngest in a family is more demanding."
> "The father is bossy. He wants more attention and must be made to realize that he is under the staff here and must do as we say."
> "I would give a wealthy person more attention because he is used to having more."

Some of these attitudes show definite evidences of biased thinking, yet these students are probably no different from some of your team members. You should try to identify your own attitudes about various people, about team nursing, and the giving of individualized patient care. Determine whether or not your attitudes are valid, since they will influence your leadership and your ability to get along with the members of your team.

PEOPLE ARE NOT ALL ALIKE

Although in many respects all human beings are similar, physically, emotionally, and spiritually, no two are exactly alike. There are differences in physical appearances, in emotional responses, and in spiritual beliefs as well as in abilities.

The Ability To Learn. People differ greatly in their ability to learn. Because of her inherent intelligence, one person may learn a great quantity of material very quickly, while another can learn only a small amount.

The mere fact that a person "learns," i.e., can repeat verbatim a certain amount of information, should not be construed to mean that she has learned it to the point of retaining it for more than a short time. Regardless of the learning process used, a certain amount of material will be forgotten and this amount will differ from person to person. Furthermore, the person who thinks of rote memorization as learning makes another serious mistake. True learning employs logical thinking and association of ideas, i.e., looking for meanings and relationships and combining them into a meaningful unit. Some people find it very easy to memorize words but find it difficult to associate ideas.

The Ability To Apply Knowledge. Closely related to the ability to see relationships and associate ideas is the ability to apply knowledge. The transference of knowledge into action is perhaps the most difficult skill a nursing student must acquire. It is easy to learn what to do in a particular situation, but change that situation ever so slightly, and the student who has only rote memory to fall back on is lost. Along with knowledge, it is also necessary to attain an understanding of basic principles and methods of applying those principles.

One morning a nursing student was assigned the care of two patients—one recovering from an appendectomy and the other suffering from a coronary thrombosis. The head nurse went over the orders for each patient but gave no further explanation to the student. Sometime later during her rounds, the head nurse found each patient giving his own bath. Calling the student aside, the head nurse asked what principle was important in the treatment of most patients suffering from heart disturbances. The student answered readily that bed rest was important for them. She had the necessary knowledge but was unable to apply it properly, for she saw no relationship between the need for bed rest and the exertion that the patient experienced in giving his own bath. To this student, bed rest was occupying a bed and nothing more.

The Ability To Use One's Hands and Body. This area includes grace, dexterity, and correct body mechanics. Some people learn readily how to make their movements graceful and effective and how to go smoothly from one motion to another. Others handle equipment and their own bodies awkwardly, with much wasted time, motion and energy. Some learn by experience, through trial and error, to achieve at least some degree of dexterity and ease of motion; other seem never to be able to attain it.

The Ability To Control or Display Emotions. To a great extent the outward show of emotion seems to be a learned behavior. The child is told, "Don't cry. You're a big girl now." So, gradually, the child learns to keep many emotions from showing outwardly. Someone says to a nursing student, "Be professional." Somewhere she acquires the idea that being professional in appearance is synonymous with acting impersonally, suppressing one's feelings in order to achieve a cool, calm, impersonal bedside manner. On the other hand, some people frequently show their emotions outwardly; some may even exaggerate them. It is possible to achieve a happy balance between the two extremes.

TEAM MEMBERS ARE PEOPLE, TOO

As you work with your team, always remember that they are individuals. You must plan for them so that their various abilities and limitations are recognized and their needs fulfilled.

STUDY QUESTIONS

1. Determine a satisfactory criterion to guide you in giving recognition and praise.
2. Do you think that the wearing of different colored uniforms by the various hospital work-groups is good? Give your reasons.
3. How could you direct your team without giving them the impression that you feel that they are working *under* you?
4. Look for situations in which a person's feelings and emotions may have affected her work.
5. What is your attitude toward each of the following? Analyze how your attitude developed. Is your attitude valid and why?
    a. A head nurse, a supervisor, a practical nurse, a nurses' aide, and a nursing student.
    b. A rich patient, and a patient from a slum district.
    c. A patient who is a Jew, a Negro, a Mexican, a Russian, or an American Indian.
    d. A patient who is a college president, a doctor, an office worker, a ditch digger, a policeman, a successful actress.
    e. A patient who is elderly, an infant, a child, a teen-ager, a young adult, a patient in his fifties.
    f. Team nursing, team leadership, team conference, nursing care plans, individualized nursing care.

3

LEADERSHIP – WHAT IS IT?

The term leadership is in itself difficult to define, since it contains broad concepts, which vary according to the person who is using the word. Sometimes it is easier to define the term by indicating the traits of a leader or the results of leadership.

SOME DEFINITIONS

Funk and Wagnalls' *Standard Dictionary* defines *leadership* as the "position of a leader; guidance," and the verb *to lead* as "to go with or ahead so as to show the way; guide."

Certainly leadership implies the presence of other people and a relationship between those people and the person who is leading. Where there is a leader there must be followers. However, mere appointment to the position of leader does not in any way insure that he will be accepted by the group, nor does it imply that he is capable of giving effective leadership. A leader must possess those qualities which enable him to make people want to accomplish something. "Leadership does not mean domination.... The leader's job is to get work done by other people, ... in getting people to work for you when they are under no obligation to do so.... No matter what point we start from in a discussion of leadership we inevitably reach the conclusion that the art of being a leader is the art of developing people."[*]

---

[*]Used with permission from *About Being a Leader* in the Monthly Letter published by the Royal Bank of Canada, October 3, 1957.

GENERAL TYPES OF LEADERSHIP

Directive Leadership. One kind of leadership is *directive*, sometimes called *autocratic*. Directive leadership in its most extreme form implies a dictator who is arbitrary and prejudiced, insisting that his is the only right way and allowing no argument, logical or otherwise, to sway him from the goal and the methods that he has selected.

In a more modified form, directive leadership combines fairness with firmness, kindliness with decisiveness, respect for the individual with power over the individual. The person using directive leadership considers himself in a position of authority, and expects his followers to respect him and to obey his directions. He may listen to suggestions, but he is not necessarily influenced by them. He has set his goals and expects them to be accepted along with his methods of achieving them. He knows what has to be accomplished and believes that he knows the best way to get it done. He does not encourage individual initiative or even cooperation between the various members of the group.

While directive leadership is not always the best form of leadership, it is necessary in cases of emergency or crisis, when there is no time for a group to decide on a plan of action. It is also useful when the leader is the only one who has new and essential information or skills, or when the members of the group are inexperienced. Also the leader must use a more directive approach when the workers expect to be told what to do, or when a worker is unsure of himself or his ability to do something on his own.

Creative Leadership. Another kind of leadership is *creative*. Here a democratic atmosphere emphasizes "togetherness." Under this form of leadership the workers are informed of the overall purposes and progress of the entire organization and of their own relationship within this organization. Each one is made to feel that he has an important contribution to make. The leader guides the workers in selecting acceptable goals and in determining an effective plan of action to achieve those goals. He allows them to make certain decisions for themselves, although he guides and helps them, consequently, they have a greater feeling of satisfaction and freedom. Creative leadership is implied in the definition, "to go with or ahead of so as to show the way."

Lao-tse, a Chinese philosopher, who lived a few hundred years before the birth of Christ, suggests that a good leader exerts his leadership in such a way that his followers do not realize that he exists, rather they believe that they did the work by themselves. The democratic leader works through people, not by domination, but by suggestion and persuasion. The more successful he is in the use of human relations, the greater is his influence as a leader.

The honor and satisfaction which he receives will not come from the public acclaim, but rather from the knowledge that his goals are reached and the work is well-done.

An extreme form of democratic leadership exists when the leader allows too much worker domination of activities with too little guidance, or when he permits the workers to do as they please until at last there is no guidance at all. This is sometimes described as "laissez faire" leadership. This let-alone policy will repudiate any leadership that may have been present at the beginning, and the work situation will rapidly disintegrate into a disorganized hodgepodge in which no one knows what he is supposed to do, nor does he care. A worker in this kind of atmosphere will lose all sense of initiative and desire for achievement. There is no place in team nursing for this kind of nonleadership.

Results of Leadership. The leader's primary purpose is to keep the group headed in the right direction. He must also decide what approach will be most effective in keeping the group constantly moving forward. But whatever the approach, effective leadership must bring results that are consistent with the aims of the organization.

While it is not easy to define leadership, it is easy to measure it in terms of what has been accomplished. Effective leadership brings several results: a spirit of cooperation and enthusiasm based on good human relationships; well-trained, skilled workers, and an efficiently run organization, able to meet its goals. In other words, good leadership improves job performance.

LEADERSHIP IN ADMINISTRATION

Leadership is needed in every area of nursing. The departmental administrator, the supervisor, the head nurse, and the staff nurse in team nursing must all be leaders, each in her particular field. The professional nurse in the hospital today is finding that she is moving away from the bedside of the patient because she must assume more and more administrative duties. This does not mean that she can become any the less concerned about patient care. It does mean that, in addition to being able to give good nursing care, she must be able to direct others in giving that care. Working with and through people is a necessary part of her leadership.

What Is Administration? Administration is the directing of a group, large or small, in its various activities so that it can reach its over-all aims in the most effective way. In any large group or organization these over-all aims are made more specific in the aims of each subdivision or department, although the point of emphasis will vary according to the specific responsibilities delegated to the department. Good administration in any area demands that definite lines of responsibility be set up through which the delegation of duties may be made along with the necessary authority to ensure their proper completion. Effective management results in the cooperation of all personnel for working toward a common goal.

An administrator is also a leader. Conversely, any leader will engage in administrative activities. An administrator guides and directs a group or an organization toward a selected goal, and a team leader becomes an administrator by virtue of the guidance and direction which she gives her team; therefore, both the administrator and the team leader must utilize the same principles in order to work with and through people.

Administrative Activities. Effective management is based upon certain principles and must be practiced by everyone who is concerned with directing people—hospital administrator, departmental administrator, supervisor, head nurse, or team leader. The scope and area of practice will be different for each of these persons, but the principles will remain the same.

Definite plans must be formulated that are based upon the objectives, policies, standards, and work procedures previously accepted by the organization. The primary objective of the hospital is caring for the patient. Every department within the hospital enlarges upon some aspect of this over-all aim. The nursing service department is concerned with giving continuous nursing care to the patient. The head nurse and her staff apply those policies, standards, and methods relating to patient care and the evaluation of that care; the team leader and her team plan ways of giving individualized patient care. By planning this care and directing the team in their work, the team leader is engaging in administrative leadership.

The plans of the organization as a whole must indicate the relationship between each department and the ways in which each must contribute to the achievement of the aims of the organization. In each case these plans must be unified and coordinated by a single individual. The team leader coordinates the activities of her team and is responsible to the head nurse, who plans and coordinates the work for a larger area. The head nurse, in turn, is responsible to the supervisor, and so on, until the final source of authority is reached.

All personnel and their activities must be systematically arranged so that responsibility and the authority for specific, well-defined duties can be delegated. The hospital organizational charts should show the direct and indirect lines of relationship, while the written policies should define clearly all duties and responsibilities. Lines of communication and the delegation of authority must follow these organizational lines over which a two-way exchange of ideas and information is of vital importance if the entire organization is to function smoothly. This two-way communication includes the administrator's responsibility for delegating functions and the worker's responsibility for reporting about her activities. Although the administrator can and should delegate duties, she cannot delegate her responsibility and must insure that all work meets acceptable standards both in quality and quantity.

The head nurse delegates certain duties to the team leader who, in turn, assigns or delegates various aspects of patient-care to her team members. She must report to her team the information and directions given to her by the head nurse, and she must keep the head nurse fully informed concerning the progress of the team in their work, referring to her any problems that she, as team leader, is unable to solve. Team members must be encouraged to go to their leader for information and help, thus allowing the team leader the opportunity to increase her administrative skill and giving the head nurse more time to function properly in her own job.

An adequate number of qualified personnel is necessary to carry out the plans and achieve the aims of the organization. The qualifications of each person will vary according to the demands of the jobs he is to do, yet each one must realize that she has a definite and important place within the framework of the organization.

To borrow a phrase from industry, "too many chiefs and not enough Indians" indicates poor administrative policies; on the other hand, a sufficient number of qualified chiefs must be available to insure good leadership for the Indians. It is impractical to insist that one group is more important than the other, for each is dependent upon the other if the goals of the organization are to be achieved. A hospital unit, if it is to give adequate care to its patients, must have sufficient administrative staff as well as other personnel who are more directly concerned with caring for the patients. However, these people with administrative responsibilities must be qualified to provide the leadership necessary for getting the work completed in an organized, effective way. On the other hand, the other workers must be qualified to perform those duties assigned to them.

As was stated previously, team nursing will not make up for a deficiency in the number of available people, but it will help to train all persons for doing their work better and, if used properly, will make more efficient use of each person. Thus, the team leader receives basic training and practical experience in the field of administration, and her team members learn how to give better nursing care.

Administration must use each person's capabilities effectively. This principle involves the use of tools of administration, such as human relations and personnel management and supervision, in order to meet the needs of the individual and to give each person adequate satisfaction in her job. Good administration considers the abilities and differences of the individual, then tries to place her in the job that best suits her capabilities. No matter how many workers are available, the work will not get done, the patients will not receive care, unless the administrator or leader is able to use each person effectively. Very little patient care will be given under the "laissez faire" form of leadership.

Frequently, all of the capabilities of an individual are not used because of inadequate planning. The administrator must know what each person can do and decide ahead of time where to place each one in order that he can do his best work. Using a worker's capabilities to the fullest extent does not mean that the administrator is a slave driver or that there is exploitation of the worker. It simply means putting the right person in the right job at the right time. Nurses frequently comment about a "well-run station" or a "poorly-run station." Undoubtedly they are referring to the results of well-planned leadership in the one instance and the apparent lack of planning and leadership in the other.

Cooperative effort is essential to coordinate the activities of the various departments and personnel. Every department and every worker contributes to the care of the patient. No one person should be allowed to consider herself more necessary or important than anyone else. Only when everyone works together harmoniously, making full use of all facilities, can the organization as a whole expect to reach its objectives. This fact is just as true for a group engaged in team nursing as it is for the hospital as a whole. The patient will benefit only to the extent that everyone gives of her abilities to help the patient. Leadership and teamwork are essential to the smooth functioning of a nursing unit.

However, someone must be responsible for planning ways and means of coordinating the care of the patient. For example, the patient will derive very little benefit if the doctor wants to start an intravenous feeding at the same time the nurses' aide wants to give the bath, the team leader wishes to irrigate a wound, and an x-ray technician wants to take an x-ray. Yet such a situation can develop if someone—head nurse or team leader—fails to plan ahead. There must be a clear understanding, however, concerning who has the final authority to do this planning. The team leader has this authority within the framework of her team, whereas the head nurse must coordinate the activities of several teams and the work of the unit as a whole.

Maximum results must be obtained with a minimum amount of time, effort, supplies, and equipment. The expenditure of money is always of great concern to administration. Economy must be practiced for the benefit of both the hospital and the patient. Unnecessary use of electricity, stationery supplies and linen, coupled with the waste of dressings, drugs, food, etc., all contribute to increased cost of hospitalization to the patient. Budgeting of supplies and care in the use of equipment must be the concern of every hospital employee.

The time and energy used by each worker must result in patient care, otherwise they are being wasted. The team leader must watch for unnecessary motions and steps and try to help her team members use their time and energy as efficiently as possible. She may need to study the causes for needless running back and forth for supplies and equipment, then plan ways for having these essentials available when and where they are needed. She may need to help a member of her team learn how to perform a certain part of a patient's care so that every motion counts.

Wasted time and effort may be dangerous, or at least annoying, to the patient. From the worker's point of view, undue effort may be so tiring that she is unable to care properly for her patients. On the other hand, undue effort by the patient as a result of nursing care awkwardly given may cause serious consequences. Every professional nurse must analyze closely the time and motions involved in giving nursing care and must look for more efficient methods. As a whole, nurses are likely to follow procedures or devise short cuts without questioning whether or not those procedures can be improved or if the short cut is safe.

Adequate reports must be made and adequate records must be kept. Records and reports contain tangible proof of the effectiveness of the activities of the group and are fundamental to good management. Well-informed people work together more efficiently, are more cooperative, and show greater interest and satisfaction in their own work and in the progress of the organization. A good report is essential for good nursing care by the individual worker, and makes administration aware of the problems as well as the progress of all the workers.

Records are written reports, indicating the work completed by the group. The patient's chart includes a report of nursing techniques performed and observations made by the staff. The head nurse is concerned with many kinds of records—the patient-condition report, census records, narcotic records, accident reports, time sheets, and others. Some records are legal documents that must be kept on file; other records are valuable for a short time only. Every department within the hospital keeps records concerning its activities. Such records are necessary if administration is to evaluate the progress of the organization.

This brief résumé of the functions of administration should make one aware that administrative and leadership skills and activities are similar. Any person who directs and supervises people must use these administrative functions. The effectiveness of their use is limited only by the capabilities of the individual and the scope of his responsibility.

LEADERSHIP IN SUPERVISION

Since administration delegates duties and responsibilities to the various departments or persons within the organization, supervision becomes a tool of administration to insure the successful completion of these duties. The supervisor must know the aims of administration and must be able to utilize effectively all administrative and leadership functions. In this way, the supervisor complements administration.

What Is Supervision? The word *supervision* conveys different ideas to different people. It is most often believed to be the inspection and checking of a worker's performance in his job by someone who looks only for those things that are being done wrong. In this conception, the emphasis of supervision is placed on getting the work done according to definite policies and procedures. The supervisor plans all the work, makes all the decisions, and issues commands to the workers who are to obey them without question. This is the traditional form of supervision, which has been practiced in industry and nursing for many years. It stifles both the initiative and the productivity of the individual and seems to think of him as a machine rather than as a human being.

Gradually, however, business and education are changing their ideas about supervision from the dictatorial to a more democratic form. The emphasis, instead of being on getting the work done, is now being placed on helping the individual do his work better. There is a greater degree of democracy and freedom, with the worker being given a voice in the setting up of work goals and planning methods for reaching them. The nursing profession is also beginning to accept these changing concepts of supervision. The implication of team nursing points to the belief that a group of people thinking, planning, and working together with competent supervision can give better nursing care than was possible under the older method of direction.

As with leadership, it is difficult to find a satisfactory definition of supervision, although it is very easy to describe the traits of a good supervisor or to determine the results of supervision. Effective supervision employs techniques from many fields of endeavor — communications, human relations, personnel management, education and others — in order to accomplish its aims. Basically, it deals with people and their personal growth; therefore, as in administration, leadership is fundamental to good supervision.

The quantity and quality of supervision will be determined by the philosophy of the individual and his ability to use the techniques on which supervision is founded. If this individual is overly directive by nature, he is likely to "drive" rather than "lead," resulting in a "do as I tell you" kind of supervision. If the person believes in creative leadership, he will make his supervision more democratic. In one, the supervision given will be direction and inspection; in the other, it will become teaching and helping the worker to develop new skills and a greater understanding of his job.

More democratic supervision is needed in nursing today, but it can be obtained only when nursing leaders believe in the worth and dignity of each person as an individual, and when they become willing to assume the responsibilities inherent in leadership, in administration and supervision. Team nursing supplies the opportunity for training more nurses in the necessary techniques and provides an unlimited field in which to practice the skills demanded by creative leadership.

Purposes of Good Supervision. Since supervision is concerned with the worker, it must also be concerned with the area where the person works — his working conditions — as well as with the work itself. The supervisor must try to provide, insofar as he is able, suitable working conditions. This involves not only the physical surroundings but also the atmosphere in which the person works. It includes the quantity of supplies and available equipment and the ease with which they can be obtained. The environment in which the person works should give him a feeling of freedom and the desire to do the best he can. The supervisor cultivates a spirit of cooperation, as evidenced by the emphasis on "we" rather than "I." Policies and procedures are formulated by the group, guided by the supervisor.

The supervisor is also concerned with the planning, the execution, and the evaluation of the work to be done. However, the worker, again guided by the supervisor, has a part in this planning and is helped to perform and evaluate his own work. On occasion, the supervisor may need to employ problem-solving techniques and experiments in order to find better methods for performing the duties delegated to his group; however, he will also seek suggestions from the members of the group.

Although the supervisor is interested in the working conditions and the work being done, his primary concern is for the

LEADERSHIP—WHAT IS IT?

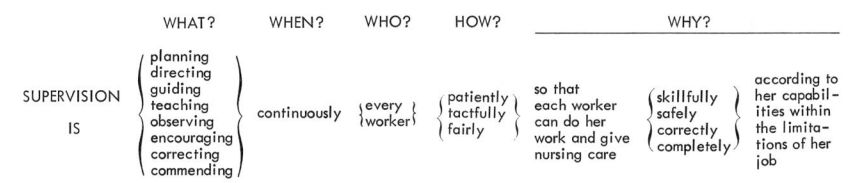

	WHAT?	WHEN?	WHO?	HOW?		WHY?
SUPERVISION IS	planning directing guiding teaching observing encouraging correcting commending	continuously	every worker	patiently tactfully fairly	so that each worker can do her work and give nursing care	skillfully safely correctly completely	according to her capabilities within the limitations of her job

Figure 1.

worker himself. One of the main aims of supervision, if not the principal one, is the orientation, training, and guidance of the individual, based upon his needs and directed toward the utilization of his capabilities and his development of new skills. The supervisor must be acquainted with each individual and be able to stimulate within each person the desire for self-improvement. Then after the person recognizes his need to improve, the supervisor must supply the necessary help and instruction, at the same time guiding the worker in the acquisition of acceptable attitudes, interests, and good work habits.

Thus, it should be apparent that administration and supervision are correlative and that the effectiveness of each depends upon the quality of leadership given to it. It seems impossible to divide these subjects into three, or even two, separate entities; rather, when one is being considered, its relation to the other must also be considered. Sometimes nursing administration, nursing supervision, and nursing leadership are spoken of as though they were three different areas of nursing endeavor or responsibility. Perhaps it would be better to think of them as interrelated activities that are part of the duties of every professional nurse.

STUDY QUESTIONS

1. Why may some people be autocratic in their direction of other people, while others are democratic?

2. Must a leader be able to perform every task better than any of the workers? State your reasons.

3. Obtain or make an organizational chart for your hospital. Trace the lines of direct and indirect relationships from the main governing body down through the various departments.

4. Determine how the main aims of your hospital are enlarged or made more specific in the objectives of each department.

5. List specific activities in team leadership in which the nurse may apply the various administrative activities.

6. Keep a record of time, supplies, and equipment that were wasted in the care of a single patient during a set interval of time. Try to estimate the cost of this waste to the patient and to the hospital. How could this waste have been avoided?

7. How are administration, supervision, and leadership similar? How do they differ?

8. What specific duties and responsibilities given to the professional nurse can she delegate to someone else? What can she not delegate?

4

LEADERSHIP IN TEAM NURSING

The team leader must always be a professional nurse. The statement that a licensed practical nurse can do anything that a registered nurse can do is misleading. Actual performance of nursing techniques cannot be the main difference between the two. The professional nurse differs from the licensed practical nurse in her ability to determine the nursing needs of each patient and to plan his care accordingly. Although the practical nurse contributes her share in caring for the patient, she is unable to judge and assess his needs. She is prepared to *assist* in giving nursing care, not to *lead*.

The word *team* implies a group of people working together cooperatively. In team nursing the group, guided by a professional nurse as leader, works together to provide individualized patient care. Cooperation and teamwork are essential in team nursing. Without leadership there can be no teamwork; on the other hand, it is possible to have leadership without teamwork. Everything depends on *how* you lead.

YOUR TYPE OF LEADERSHIP— DIRECTIVE OR CREATIVE?

Your method of leadership will vary according to the existing situation and may change from day to day, even from hour to hour.

LEADERSHIP IN TEAM NURSING

Your team members will be watching you, listening to you, deciding how they feel about you. Their decision will be based upon your ability to put your leadership across. If they feel ignored, not part of the team, or necessary only to get the work done, you may find yourself a leader in name only.

Suppose that one morning you have a new and inexperienced aide assigned to your team. Remember that first impressions are often lasting impressions. It is important that your leadership start from the moment she becomes a part of your group. You must make her feel that she is needed, for with that feeling comes the desire to participate and cooperate in the team's activities. Introducing yourself and the other members of the group is important. It is also important that she recognize that you are the one to whom she can come for help. You will probably want to use directive leadership at first, since she is new in the hospital situation and is likely to be unsure of herself. Make sure that she understands her duties — what she is to do, when, and how; to whom she is to report, and why. It is never wise to allow another worker of the same rank to be responsible for this period of orientation.

An emergency arises — a patient's condition suddenly becomes critical, an accident case is admitted in the middle of a busy morning. Your team will look to you for instructions about what to do; again you will use directive leadership. Decisions must be made immediately — what to do, how to do it, and who is best qualified. Everyone works together, but you give specific directions. You are the leader — the one who knows the way. Yet when the emergency is past, you did not meet it alone; you and your team met it together. This is the result of leadership. Remember to give credit for cooperation and for a job done well together.

These are only two examples of situations in which you will find that directive leadership is necessary; there will be others. In each case you will use the method of leadership that best meets the needs of your team members and the needs of your patients.

As you gain experience, your leadership can become more democratic or creative. You should recognize the contribution that each person is capable of making toward meeting the needs of the patients, and you should encourage each person to obtain a greater understanding of nursing care. As your team gains this understanding, you should give them more opportunities to suggest ways of meeting various patient care problems, rather than telling them how. You should encourage each one to participate in the planning of patient care. This does not mean that your leadership will become less. Actually, your leadership should become greater than before, for you must continually seek ways in which you and your team can improve the nursing care of your patients. Remember that the quality of nursing care, the quality of team play, the quality

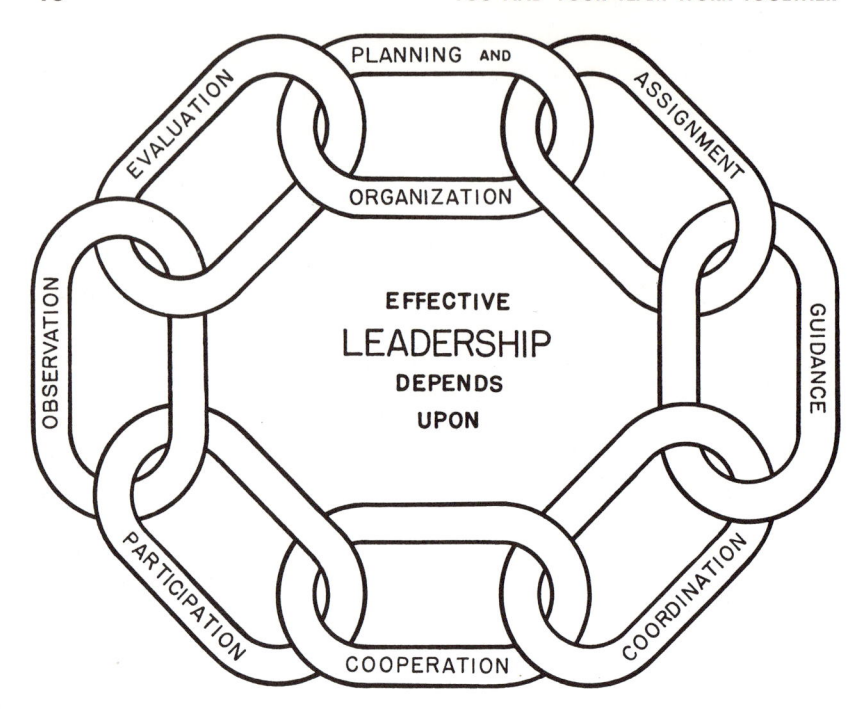

Figure 2. *Leadership is only as strong as the weakest link in this chain.*

of respect for each person as an individual will be no greater than you demonstrate in your leadership. These concepts provide the challenge of creative leadership in team nursing.

TECHNIQUES OF TEAM LEADERSHIP

First of all, you must be a firm believer in the principles of team nursing, as well as be aware of and willing to accept the responsibilities of team leadership. You must know each of your team members, recognizing each person's needs and differences as individuals. You must be able to help each one satisfy her needs. You will need to make allowances for her different abilities, attitudes, feelings and emotions. You must understand the principles and techniques employed in administration and supervision, as well as those employed in giving nursing care, for your leadership must be guided by these principles and techniques. For example, you will not be concerned with making out hours for the staff on the station, but you will be, or should be, concerned with making the best use of your team's time and energy. You may not be concerned with the ordering of supplies for use by the entire station, but you will certainly be concerned about seeing that the supplies used by your team are not wasted.

Planning and Organizing. Plan and organize your own work. Coordinate all team activities so that everything gets done at the proper time and in the correct way. Perhaps you have had the unhappy experience of working with a person who "flits" from one job to another; makes frequent trips to get equipment and supplies, which she forgot to bring with her the first time; neglects to remind someone to do something until it is too late; works too fast; talks too fast; and looks hurried and breathless. Soon those who work with her look and act the same way. The patients feel the pressure and, although they may not realize exactly why, they are not comfortable or relaxed. These are the results of disorganization.

On the other hand, you may know a nurse who, when an emergency arises, does not seem to move any faster or raise her voice. People can be rushing around frantically, yet, when she takes charge, everyone seems to relax. Order is restored, and the work is done quickly in an orderly fashion. How is she able to accomplish this? Does she possess some magic? No, but she is a leader who thinks and acts in a systematic way. There is never any wasted motion. She knows what to do and the most efficient way to do it. However, she did not acquire this ability overnight. It came with her learning how to plan and organize, first, her work as a nursing student, and later, her more complex duties as a graduate nurse.

Making Assignments and Giving Directions. Regardless of the method used in making assignments in team nursing in your hospital, you will be giving directions; therefore, you must be able to plan ahead and give those directions clearly and concisely. They may be as simple as asking a nurses' aide to take a glassful of water to a patient or as complicated as making and explaining patient assignments to your team. In either case, you must make the individual understand the directions you are giving. You are also responsible for determining whether the task is completed in the proper way. You will need to work with people who have varying degrees of experience and knowledge, from the freshman nursing student or inexperienced nurses' aide to the experienced practical nurse or even the professional nurse. You will need to use all your knowledge and understanding of human relations and nursing techniques.

Guidance. Guidance is a valuable tool in the hands of the team leader. The word *guidance* implies going before, leading the way, and makes use of various teaching and counseling methods. In addition to having a thorough knowledge of nursing and its many skills, you must have the ability to help each member of your team perform her assigned duties both to her own satisfaction and to the satisfaction of the patient.

This does not mean that you will become a counselor in the usual sense of the word. It does, however, mean that you must recognize the relationship of personal problems and emotions to the ability of the individual to do a good job. It also means that, by example, you will demonstrate what you expect of your team in giving nursing care and understanding to the patient.

Cooperation. You must cooperate with and encourage cooperation among your team members. Leadership is essential if you are to have teamwork. The amount of cooperation that exists within your team will depend greatly upon you and your attitude toward them as individuals. Remember that they are working *with* you, not *for* or *under* you. The idea of subservience, indicated by the words *for* and *under*, implies extreme directive leadership and stifles the feeling of cooperation essential to the effective practice of team nursing.

Cooperation is encouraged by an atmosphere of democracy in which the individual knows what is expected of her, is kept informed of her progress, and is stimulated to improve through the praise and constructive criticism skillfully given by the leader. Let your team know that you have confidence in them. Do not ask them to do something which you would not be willing to do yourself. Say "will you" more often than "you must." Good human relations stimulate cooperation and loyalty among your team members.

Encouraging Participation. You should provide opportunities for the participation of each team member in team activities. Working with a group fosters the feeling of belonging to that group. Participation may take various forms, depending upon the person's abilities and desires. It does not imply merely talking at team conferences or doing a certain amount of work, although these are certainly desirable forms of participation. Cooperation is closely allied to participation; both must be active rather than passive.

You will need to provide obvious opportunities for the cooperation and participation by the individual who tends to be withdrawn and passive. Recognition for her participation is important to her. Even though she may be wrong, for example, giving information that is incomplete or incorrect during a discussion, you should recognize her contribution, although you will need to correct her.

Coordination. Coordination of activities within the nursing team, and between your team and other personnel, is a necessary part of team leadership. You need to keep your team informed about the various ward and hospital activities. Also you need to report to your head nurse or supervisor about the work accomplished by your team. You will want to utilize the services of other people or agencies, thereby making all of the hospital and community resources available to the patient. You will need to plan to prevent conflicts in the performance of duties as your team members go about their work. Coordination is based upon good planning and the utilization of the abilities of each member of your team and the resources found within the hospital and surrounding community.

Observation. The observation of your team and their work is one of your biggest responsibilities as team leader. Observation must be more than just checking and inspecting; it is the acquisition of knowledge through the use of all of your senses. You need to be able to see nursing care in its entirety as well as its individual aspects. To do this you will need to observe not only the physical performance of the worker but also the manifestations of those abstract areas involving her emotions and understanding.

Evaluation. Not only must you learn to observe correctly, but you must also learn to evaluate your observations. Evaluation should be a continuous process of analyzing the strengths and the weaknesses that you observe in the personnel themselves or in their work, so that you can encourage them to continue doing good work or help them to improve in those areas in which they are weak. To be able to analyze fairly, you must set up some definite goals beforehand and have direct personal contact with the persons and the work you want to evaluate; otherwise, you have nothing on which you can base your judgment.

You must also evaluate yourself, as a person, as a nurse, and as a leader; for, if you are unable to criticize yourself honestly, you have no right to criticize others. This ability to do self-evaluation is one of the attributes that every leader must develop.

But after evaluation, what? Is your work finished? By no means! After determining your progress as a team and where you need to improve, you will need to set new goals, make new plans, reorganize your resources, and begin work again. Leadership can never become static; for, when it rests on past achievements, there is no longer any leadership.

THE IMPORTANCE OF EFFECTIVE COMMUNICATION

In order to get along with people, we must be able to communicate with them and make ourselves clearly understood. Communication is necessary to use the techniques of leadership. The more effective a leader's communication, the more effective will be her leadership.

What Is Communication? Communication is more than just saying words. It is the ability to convey ideas and meanings to another person. We have all heard the saying, "Your actions speak so loudly, I can't hear what you say." So it is with our communication. What we do and how we do it convey just as much meaning as what we say; in fact, *what* we say may be less important than *how* we say it. The tone of voice, choice of word, facial expressions and gestures may communicate our ideas and feelings more effectively sometimes than the actual words we use.

To be really effective, communication must be an interchange of ideas. What we say is less important than what people think we are saying; we must make certain that we are putting our ideas across. Not only must we try to make ourselves understood but we must also be open-minded, trying to understand others and their ideas and suggestions.

Communication may be either directive or creative. It is directive when the team leader assigns duties, gives definite information, or demonstrates how to perform a procedure. She uses creative communication when she helps a team member determine what should be done and how to do it, or when she listens to someone talk over a personal problem.

How Do We Communicate? Good communication begins with a clear idea about what one wants to say and how to say it. The English language is very complex; a single word may have many meanings, sometimes similar, sometimes dissimilar. A classic example of this is the difference in the meaning that the word *void* conveys to a bookkeeper and to a nurse. *Normal* has a different meaning for a chemist than it does for a biologist, a mathematician, or a psychologist. The word *careful* has at least eight different shades of meaning, while the word *see* has at least twenty. The context of the sentence may indicate the meaning of the word, or the meaning may be inferred from the inflection of the speaker's voice.

As in every profession or trade, hospital workers have their own terminology and jargon, which are, for the most part, extremely puzzling to the uninitiated. Nursing students and new aides quickly pick up this new language and use it as a badge of belonging. Thus cath., prep., O.R., I.V., I.M., trach. care, E.K.G., ad lib, and many others creep into the conversation with patients as well as with other hospital personnel. It seems so easy for the nurse to say to a patient, "Have you been preped for your g.i. studies tomorrow?" In fact, one nursing student went so far as to chart, "Pt. went to B.R. for B.M. before the lab came to do her B.M.R."

Certain terms and abbreviations are acceptable; however, we should never overuse them nor include them in our conversations with patients. Terminology that seems very commonplace to us can be confusing and frightening to the patient. We must be able to select the word that not only conveys our meaning in the best way, but is also one which is familiar to our listeners. If a word is unfamiliar, then we must define it in terms that the listener can understand.

Not only is communication carried on through the use of words but also by means of the tone or inflection of the voice. For example, take the simple word *yes*. By changing the inflection one may express simple agreement, agreement and sympathy, question, disgust or irritation, ridicule, or astonishment. In addition, gestures and facial expressions convey information about one's feelings. Nodding one's head may indicate agreement, interest, and/or sympathy; raising an eyebrow may show doubt. Words do not need to be used in order to communicate with others.

Another method of conveying ideas is by means of the written word. We communicate through written assignments, reports, and charts. Belonging to a profession implies a certain quality and quantity of education. Yet professional nurses sometimes demonstrate a surprising lack of knowledge about correct grammar and spelling.

As stated previously, facial expressions and gestures convey ideas. In like manner, the use of visual aids to illustrate the ideas we are trying to put across is an effective means of communication. The demonstration of a certain technique or procedure is much more effective than a verbal description only. Put the two together and it becomes easier to put the idea across.

What we do is observed by others. Our actions demonstrate our attitudes and depths of understanding more effectively than all the talking we do. Those who work with us will judge our actions and assume that, since we are professional nurses, the way in which we do our work must be the correct and best way.

You must remember that good communication is necessary for understanding and for cooperation and unified action. Communication, to be effective, must move toward you as well as from you. You must be able to put yourself and your ideas across. On the other hand, you must provide the opportunity for, and seek to understand, communication by others.

How Well Do We Try To Understand Others? Most of us have a tendency to talk too much and listen too little. When trying to find out what others think and believe, we should try to keep our questions and comments brief and to the point. As the old jingle puts it:

> A wise old owl lived in an oak.
> The more he saw, the less he spoke;
> The less he spoke, the more he heard.
> Why can't we be like that wise old bird?

In order to understand others, we must learn to listen with an open mind. To do this we must learn to control our feelings and opinions and become more receptive to those of others. We often think and judge with our feelings; therefore, we must guard against reading our own meaning into what the other person is saying. We cannot afford to jump to a hasty conclusion.

In addition, if we want to understand what we hear, we must be genuinely interested in the other person and in what she is saying. We can display that interest by our expressions, questions, and comments; interest is also shown by our providing the opportunity for others to express themselves.

The ability to understand what another person is saying goes far beyond the recognition of the words used. It involves trying to understand any display of emotions, attitudes, or prejudices. In addition, it means recognizing that what a person does not say may be as important as what he does say. It is only natural for us to try to "save face" and to protect our egos from being undermined. Therefore, we are likely to sound out those around us to determine whether they will be sympathetic and understanding or critical of our actions, opinions, attitudes, or beliefs. Sometimes we are totally unaware that we are using this method of self-protection. For example, a nurses' aide may remark to the team leader, "Mr. Smith seems to feel that he can't ask the nurses to help him." Could it be that she also has that feeling but is transferring it to a third person to find out what the nurse's reaction might be? Perhaps, if we show more interest in and sympathy for our patients, the team members will feel freer to ask for help or to express their opinions and ideas.

Common Barriers to Good Understanding. Probably the most common cause of misunderstanding is found in our own preconceived ideas, opinions, and beliefs. We are sometimes unable to evaluate facts objectively, because we interpret them with our feelings in the light of our past experience. In doing so we may use false logic. For example, we may believe that:

People who are shifty-eyed do not tell the truth.—Major premise.

Mary Jones is shifty-eyed.—Minor premise.

Therefore, Mary Jones is not telling the truth.—Conclusion.

Our major premise is based upon our belief, which is not a proven fact; therefore, our conclusion may be incorrect. However, our dislike of Mary Jones has begun and, regardless of the circumstances, which may later disprove our original opinion of her, we will have difficulty in overcoming this prejudice. Furthermore, we may communicate our distrust through our actions, and the barrier to mutual understanding grows higher.

Another reason for misunderstanding is found in the fact that

LEADERSHIP IN TEAM NURSING **47**

we are prone to judge in terms of either right or wrong with no degrees in between. This interpretation is based, as was previously indicated, on our own opinions, ideas, and beliefs, rather than on research and critical analysis of all the available facts. Sometimes we do not even attempt to discover all the facts, or perhaps we are unable or unwilling to consider anyone's viewpoint but our own.

We sometimes behave like the six blind men in the Hindoo fable. Each went to find out for himself what an elephant looked like. The first man felt the side and decided that the animal was like a wall. The next man happened to feel the tusk, so he was sure that the elephant was like a spear. Still another grabbed the trunk, so he thought the animal was like a snake. The fourth blind man put his arms around the elephant's leg; consequently, to him, the animal was like a tree. The next man felt the elephant's ear, so he compared the animal to a fan. Finally, the last one seized the tail and immediately he thought the elephant was like a rope. Each of the six men clung to his own opinion of what the elephant looked like. Although each man was partly right, each one thought his opinion was the only correct one, and all others were wrong; therefore, no one made any further attempt to find out the truth.

We arrange words into sentences to express ideas. When our grammar is faulty, we have difficulty saying what we mean. The ability of others to understand what we say is, at least in part, dependent upon our ability to place words in their correct relationship to one another. Dangling phrases and indefinite reference or agreement of pronouns will confuse the listener. For example, "having sterilized the instruments, the operation was started" is confusing to say the least. Or suppose you are given this direction, "I'll hold his knee, and when I nod my head, tap it." Would you do as you are told? Using the English language correctly is a necessary part of effective communication.

If we are to be understood, we must speak the language of our listeners. The dangers of misunderstanding arising out of our indiscriminate use of medical terminology and hospital jargon have already been discussed. The mark of an educated person is his ability to speak the language of those around him. Sometimes our desire to demonstrate our knowledge of a subject leads us to use difficult words and lengthy explanations; consequently, what we are saying does not mean much to our listeners. The simpler we make our language, the more likely we are to be understood.

The use of abstract terms and ideas in place of specific words and definitions is still another reason for misunderstandings. Perhaps we are mentally lazy; at any rate, we do not always define clearly in our own minds just what we are trying to say; therefore, others do not understand us well. Abstract terms will be given more concrete meanings by the other person. Thus *small* may mean a drop, a part of a teaspoonful, an entire teaspoonful, a pinch, one piece, a number of pieces, and so on. *Some, large,* a *few* minutes, *don't overdo,* and *just routine* are examples of abstract words and phrases that may mean different things to different people.

Other factors also contribute to our being misunderstood. The listener must be interested if he is to grasp the entire meaning. We can never assume that our listener understands what we are saying. We must always watch for the puzzled expression or frown and try to clarify the point immediately to the satisfaction of all concerned.

How Can You Communicate More Effectively? Think before you speak. Determine what you want to say and how you can say it so that it will be easily understood by others. Be brief and choose your words with care; make each one count.

Mean what you say. Remember that your tone of voice, facial expression, and actions must be in harmony with the content of your message, emphasizing its meaning rather than detracting from it. Put the message in personal terms directed for the personal use of the listener. However, you must talk *with* rather than *at,* and certainly never *down to,* your listener. The pronoun, *I,* should be used less often than *we.* The pronoun, *you,* encourages personal application by directive suggestion, whereas *we* suggests togetherness or belonging. When used properly, each pronoun can contribute to putting across your ideas more effectively.

State your facts objectively. However, you must keep in mind the importance of the other person's emotions in relation to what you are saying. Whenever possible, use a combination of methods of communication—visual as well as verbal—in order to emphasize what you say. Define key terms, then follow with illustrations that are familiar to your listener. Always start with the familiar and proceed to the unknown. Choose definite and specific words rather than abstract ones. In addition, keep in mind the importance of understanding others. Try to evaluate objectively all that you see and hear.

The Art of Gentle Persuasion. We can see the use of persuasion all around us every day. Advertising is one of the most common forms. Teaching also uses persuasion. The books and newspapers we read, the pictures we look at, the conversations we engage in— most, if not all, are directed toward persuading us more or less subtly to believe something and to translate our beliefs into action.

Persuasion is an important activity in leadership, for through persuasion you get a person to do or to believe something because she wants to do or to believe it. Listening is one of the first steps in persuasion. Find out what a person believes and why she believes it. Don't argue or contradict. Ask one or two questions to

LEADERSHIP IN TEAM NURSING

which the person can answer "Yes." Make one or two suggestions. Avoid those words suggesting ideas against which she has already indicated prejudice. Make your ideas attractive. Show the person how much she will benefit from following your ideas. (This is a basic principle in advertising. "Feel good again with . . . tonic!" or "Want to look your best? Wear a . . . girdle.") Later, the person may offer your original idea as if it was hers from the very beginning. This is the result of effective persuasion. Now she will believe in that idea because it is hers.

Rumors and What To Do about Them. Almost always rumors are caused by a lack of communication. Much has been said about the hospital grapevine. When people feel that they have not been told everything, they will quickly supply their own reasons. Sometimes they would rather believe a false statement than a true one, because it is what they want to believe. Rumors are also caused by a misunderstanding somewhere along the line of communication or by the prejudices and personal opinions of a listener.

Preventing rumors is better than trying to stop them after they have been started; therefore, you must keep your team well-informed concerning changes in hospital policies and the reasons for these changes. No rumor should be ignored, for it indicates that the line of communication has become blocked somewhere. Get all the available facts and pass them on to your team as soon as possible.

DO YOU HAVE WHAT IT TAKES TO BE A LEADER?

Qualities Needed by a Leader. A team leader must possess certain definite qualities. First of all, she must be a professional nurse in every sense of the word. She must be willing to assume those responsibilities concomitant with her profession. Not only must she know what constitutes good nursing care but also she must give good care to her patients. She must be interested in people and be able to communicate with them effectively.

Good health is very necessary, for it is closely related to emotions and influences, to a great extent, how the nurse feels about her work and toward those with whom she is working.

A leader must also be a follower. This may sound contradictory, yet the democratic leader helps her team to decide what should be done and is guided by their suggestions. In team nursing especially, there must be united effort and a constant interchange of ideas.

One of the most important qualities for the team leader is

emotional maturity. This kind of maturity has nothing to do with physical age; rather, it implies that the individual has reached a stage in her development when she has become independent in thought and action, with the ability to make decisions based on her analysis of all available facts. The mature person is more concerned with others than with herself; she thinks more about giving than getting. She does not dwell on the past and its errors, although she uses the lessons learned through them to improve herself. She has learned to criticize herself objectively and is flexible enough to try to change those personal characteristics that she feels are not consistent with what she wants to be. She has also learned that she is only human and, therefore, not perfect; consequently, she tries to be tolerant of others, abhorring the faults but not the individual. She strives to be consistent and fair in all her dealings.

Leadership is not free; it demands the price of great mental and physical effort, of more self-criticism, self-control, and self-confidence. In fact, Eleanor C. Lambertsen* maintains that "a primary factor in successful leadership is the leader's belief in the philosophy of the nursing team, and in the confidence she feels in her ability as a leader."

What Do Team Members Want in a Leader? In a questionnaire answered by a number of nurses' aides, 55 per cent listed personal characteristics such as kindness and understanding as being the most important qualities of a leader. Another 40 per cent thought that a thorough knowledge of the work to be done was most important. The characteristic that 70 per cent of these aides indicated they disliked most was the unwillingness or inability of the team leader to give help or advice.

In answer to the question "How can your team leader help you more?" 95 per cent wanted more help in learning how to do their work. They indicated this help could be given by answering their questions, teaching them how to care for their patients, or by giving them more information about their patients.

Take a Self-inventory. What qualities do you consider most important in a leader? How well do you measure up to those qualities? What are your weakest points? Oh, come now, you must have some. Where do you need to improve? What can you do about it?

Write down some goals for yourself. Don't be too ambitious at first. Perhaps you resolve to show more interest in others. That is a good objective, but it is also a very hard one to attain. Why not select one or two actions that demonstrate this quality and resolve

---

*Lambertsen, Eleanor C.: *Nursing Team — Organization and Functioning.* Published for the Division of Nursing Education by the Bureau of Publications, Teachers College, Columbia, 1953, page 22.

LEADERSHIP IN TEAM NURSING **51**

to practice them whenever possible. How many times do you use *I, me,* or *mine* in your conversation instead of *you, yours, we* or *us*? Do you sometimes say something to a person then suddenly realize that you could have been more tactful? Why not do your wondering before you speak? Whatever it is that you resolve to change, select a number of aspects and concentrate on them.

Now put your resolutions into action—today, everyday, in every way that you possibly can. Always keep them in mind. Think of them every morning and again every night. Maybe you'll fail a time or two. Don't give up; keep trying.

At regular intervals sit down and add up your score. So you didn't do as well as you had hoped. Try to find out where and why you failed. Were you positive in your attitude and approach or did you become discouraged easily when you discovered that you could not miraculously reach your goal overnight? Try again—and again—and again. This is the price you have to pay if you want to become an effective team leader.

STUDY QUESTIONS

1. What do you mean when you use the following expressions: in a minute, don't worry, just a routine specimen, "clean" and "dirty" cases, float nurse, scrub nurse, neurotic? How might each expression be interpreted by a patient, by a freshman nursing student, by an inexperienced nurses' aide?

2. Observe the hospital ward for illustrations of communications (verbal and nonverbal) that were or could have been misunderstood by one of the persons involved. What should be done to improve the communication?

3. Make a list of abstract words or phrases that a nurse commonly uses. How can each be made more specific in meaning?

4. Trace one rumor. Determine, if possible, its cause and how it could have been prevented.

5. Observe situations illustrating directive leadership and creative leadership. If you do not agree with the type of leadership used in each situation, give your reasons.

6. Compare team leadership techniques with administrative and supervisory activities.

7. How can team leadership prepare the nurse for an administrative position?

8. What qualities and personal characteristics do you consider most important in a team leader?

PART TWO BIBLIOGRAPHY

Books

Dennis, Lorraine Bradt: *Psychology of Human Behavior for Nurses.* W. B. Saunders Company, Philadelphia, 1962.
Dooher, M. Joseph, Editor, and Marquis, Vivienne, Associate Editor: *Effective Communication on the Job.* American Management Association, New York, 1956.

Flesch, Rudolf: *The Art of Plain Talk.* Harper Bros., New York, 1946.
Gardiner, Glenn, et al: *Managerial Skills for Supervisors.* Elliot Service Company, Mount Vernon, N. Y., 1960.
Laird, Donald C., and Laird, Eleanor C.: *Practical Business Psychology.* McGraw-Hill Book Company, New York, 1961.
Lambertsen, Eleanor C.: *Nursing Team: Organization and Functioning.* Published for the Division of Nursing Education by the Bureau of Publications, Teacher's College, Columbia University, 1953.
Leadership on the Job. Edited by the staff of Supervisory Management, American Management Association, New York, 1957.
Newcomb, Dorothy Perkins: *The Team Plan, A Manual for Nursing Service Administrators.* G. P. Putnam's Sons, Inc., New York, 1953.
Osborn, Alex F.: *Applied Imagination.* Charles Scribner's Sons, New York, 1957.
Perrodin, Cecilia M.: *Supervision of Nursing Service Personnel.* The Macmillan Company, New York, 1957.
Pieper, Frank: *Modular Management and Human Leadership.* Methods Press, Minneapolis, 1958.
Saxe, John Godfrey: *The Blind Men and the Elephant.* Home Book of Verse, edited by B. E. Stevenson, Vol. 1, page 1877. Henry Holt & Company, Inc., 1940.
Tead, Ordway: *The Art of Leadership.* McGraw-Hill Book Company, Inc., New York, 1935.
Uris, Auren: *Techniques of Leadership.* McGraw-Hill Book Company, Inc., New York, 1953.

Journals

About Being a Leader. Monthly Letter of the Royal Bank of Canada, Montreal, Oct. 3, 1957.
Are We Nursing the Patients—or the Paper Work? RN, 27:12:54, Dec., 1964.
Building Morale for Better Job Performance. Jobber Executive, Hunter Publishing Company, Chicago, July, 1965, page 22.
Coletti, Angela C.: *The Head Nurse Is a Manager.* Hospital Progress. 41:3:100, March, 1960.
Corona, Dorothy F.: *Sedatives and Stimulants to Creativity.* Nurs. Outlook, 12: 7:24, July, 1964.
Cline, Dorothy S.: *An Analysis of Spelling Errors Made by Professional Nurses.* Nurs. Outlook, 7:7:400, July, 1959.
Crosby, Edwin L.: *Coordination or Fragmentation?* Nurs. Outlook, 11:1:42, Jan., 1963.
Davis, Anne J.: *The Skills of Communication.* Am. J. Nursing, 63:1:66, Jan., 1963.
Davis, Keith: *Good Listener, Good Nurse.* RN, 26:10:113, Oct., 1963.
DeArmond, Fred: *How to Put Your Ideas Across.* RN, 21:12:63, Dec., 1958.
Dennis, Robert J.: *Ways of Caring.* Am. J. Nursing, 64:2:107, Feb., 1964.
Dunn, Helen: *Good Communication/Good Administration.* Nurs. Outlook, 9:11: 670, Nov., 1961.
Elder, Ruth G.: *What Is the Patient Saying?* Nursing Forum, 2:1:24, July, 1963.
Gerard, Richard W.: *The Importance of Communication.* Hospital Management, 89:5:73, May, 1960.
Gilbreth, Lillian: *The Basic Questions of Management.* Hospital Progress, 42:1:55, Jan., 1961.
How to Improve Job Performance Through Good Leadership. Management Course for Air Force Supervisors, Air Force Pamphlet No. 50-2-25, United States Government Printing Office, Washington, D.C., June, 1955.
Jackson, Joan K.: *Communication Is Important.* Am. J. Nursing, 59:1:90, Jan., 1959.
Johnson, Betty Sue: *The Meaning of Touch in Nursing.* Nurs. Outlook, 13:2:59, Feb., 1965.
Lagemann, John Kord: *Your Words Give You Away.* Reader's Digest, 79:17, Aug., 1961.
Leino, Amelia: *Organizing the Nursing Team.* Am. J. Nursing, 51:11:665, Nov., 1951.

Leone, Lucile Petry: *Accent on Leadership.* Am. J. Nursing, 58:10:1419, Oct., 1958.
Margarella, Sister Mary: *Communication: The Catalyst.* Hospital Progress, 41:5: 106, May, 1960.
Miller, Mary Annice: *Essentials for Self and Staff Improvement.* Am. J. Nursing. 61:11:85, Nov., 1961.
Newton, Mildred E.: *Developing Leadership Potential.* Nurs. Outlook, 5:7:400, July, 1957.
Neylan, Margaret Prowse: *Anxiety.* Am. J. Nursing, 62:5:110, May, 1962.
O'Donovan, Thomas R.: *Effective Supervision Requires Leadership.* Hospital Progress, Feb., 1965, page 65.
Oshin, Edith S.: *How to Argue without Losing Your Head.* RN, 25:10:81, Oct., 1962.
Paulsen, Dorothy: *Patients Give Tests Too.* Am. J. Nursing, 62:8:58, Aug., 1962.
Paynich, Mary Louise: *Cultural Barriers to Nurse Communication.* Am. J. Nursing, 64:2:87, Feb., 1964.
Perkins, Ralph: *The Do's and Don'ts of Delegation.* Hospitals, 36:17:40, Sept., 1962.
Polacci, Sister Margaret Mary: *Process Recording by Staff Nurses.* Nurs. Outlook, 11:7:530, July, 1963.
Pollock, Ted: *Put Your Ideas Across—Effectively.* Hospital Management, 99:5:68, May, 1965.
Robinson, Alice M.: *Creativity Takes Courage.* Nurs. Outlook. 11:7:499, July, 1963.
Rockwell, F. A.: *Writers are Not Spiders.* Author & Journalist, 49:1:12, Feb., 1964.
Roth, Julius A.: *How Nurses' Aides Learn Their Jobs.* Am. J. Nursing, 62:8:54, Aug., 1962.
Sells, Annabell C.: *The First Line Supervisors and Human Relations.* Canadian Nurse, 61:4:283, April, 1965.
Siggins, Clara M.: *A Professor of English Looks at Communication Skills.* Nurs. Outlook, 9:11:666, Nov., 1961.
Skipper, James K., et al: *Some Barriers to Communication.* Nursing Forum, 2:1:14, July, 1963.
Smith, Carol Anne: *Job Satisfaction in Hospital Nursing.* Canadian Nurse, 59:2:147, Feb., 1963.
Smith, Dorothy M.: *The Nursing Team: Fact or Fancy.* Minnesota Nursing Accent, Minnesota Nurses' Association, St. Paul, 36:2:26, Feb., 1964.
Stander, Norman E.: *Basic Elements of Reliability Training.* Personnel, 41:1:70, Jan.-Feb., 1964.
The Art of Supervision. Social Security Administration, Division of Management, United States Government Printing Office, Washington, D.C., Jan., 1964
The "Seven Deadly Sins" of Supervisors. Jobber Executive, Hunter Publishing Company, Chicago, May, 1965, page 21.
Villeneuve, Jacques P.: *Development of Human Resources.* Canadian Nurse, 61:2:94, Feb., 1965.
Willard, Marian C.: *A Matter of Facts.* Nurs. Outlook, 11:11:832, Nov., 1963.
Winslow, John: *How's Your Talent for "Taking Charge"?* RN, 25:4:62, April, 1962.
Witt, John A.: *Good Communication or a Partial Vacuum.* Hospitals, 36:16:51, Aug. 16, 1962.
Wolfe, Ilse: *What's in a Word?* Nurs. Outlook, 12:12:36, Dec., 1964.
Wood, M. Marian: *From General Duty Nurse to Team Leader.* Am. J. Nursing, 63:1:104, Jan., 1963.
Yancey, Donna: *Without Words.* Am. J. Nursing, 62:11:118, Nov., 1962.

_____ PART THREE

How To Lead Your Team

*I keep six honest serving-men
    (They taught me all I knew);
Their names are What and Why and When
    and How and Where and Who.*

                    from The Elephant's Child, Stanza I,
                              by Rudyard Kipling

5

HOW TO ORGANIZE YOUR WORK

If you are to become a good team leader, you must learn how to use the techniques of leadership, administration and supervision intelligently in many different situations. For this reason, Part Three is devoted to a discussion of the various ways in which you may apply these principles in the leadership of your team.

HOW TO PREPARE YOURSELF

What Is Necessary for Effective Organization? In order to accomplish anything you must first have a plan. Planning means constantly thinking ahead and deciding on a course of action. Organization is only one aspect of planning and is the orderly arrangement of related activities according to time and importance.

KNOWLEDGE IS NECESSARY FOR GOOD PLANNING. Since part of the aim of team nursing is to give patient-centered care, you must become acquainted with the patient as an individual and become aware of his problems. You must also have the necessary knowledge and skill to give the kind of care that his condition and problems demand. You may have a nursing care plan already available; however, if you are in the process of instituting team nursing, or if you have recently admitted patients for whom care plans have not yet been developed, you will need to visit your patients in order to get enough information to help plan your work.

You must also know what is expected of you as a team leader. Since each hospital adapts the principles of team nursing to fit its own needs and situation, you must learn what duties, responsibilities, and authority have been delegated to you by the supervisor and head nurse of your unit. You will need to learn as much as you can about hospital policies and routines, both written and unwritten, and keep yourself informed concerning changes as they are made. Various ways may be used to inform you of these policies and changes; for example, the hospital policy book, the ward manual (sometimes called the secretary's manual or head nurse's manual), written memoranda posted on the bulletin board, verbal reports by the head nurse or supervisor, or the in-service educational program.

As team leader you will need to have some definite information about your team members, not only about the duties to which they may be assigned but also about their abilities and limitations as individuals. Job descriptions can usually be found in the hospital policy book or similar manual. As you become acquainted with your team, you will gain a more complete understanding of each person, her likes, dislikes, aptitudes, and attitudes. When planning the work of your team, you should use this personal information in order to coordinate and complement the abilities of each worker. For example, you may assign a person who moves quickly but has a tendency to omit small details to work with a person who moves more slowly and gives greater attention to details. On the other hand, if there is a personality clash between two individuals, you will destroy the spirit of teamwork and cooperation if you assign these two to work together.

PLANNING IS NECESSARY FOR EFFECTIVE ACTION. When there is no plan, only confusion exists. Planning implies knowing where you are going, and it is necessary if you are to learn how to get there. Without this knowledge, all activity will be so haphazard that little will be accomplished. In the leadership of the nursing team, planning and organization are essential not only to provide good nursing care but also to promote cooperation. Organization is necessary if each individual is to gain an understanding of what is expected of her. With this understanding comes a feeling of greater security, essential for job satisfaction and better job performance.

Relationship of Problem-solving to Planning. Planning is solving problems, or better, foreseeing certain problems and preventing their occurrence. Even though you may have planned your work carefully, situations sometimes develop that you must straighten out. Your team members recognize that problems may occur. They want a leader who thinks before she speaks or acts, one who will help them in a systematic way.

Systematic thinking, sometimes called the "scientific method" of thinking, can be done by using the five steps of problem-solving. You have probably used these steps before, or at least some of them, but do you know them well enough so that you can use them consciously to solve or prevent problems which you and your team may encounter?

IDENTIFY AND DEFINE THE PROBLEM. Perhaps an incident occurs that necessitates action on your part. In many cases the incident itself is not the main problem; rather it is the result of one or more difficulties already existing. It may help you to identify them if you ask yourself, "Why?" or "What?" When you find these underlying causes, you can concentrate on the problem, or several aspects of it, in order to eliminate the major issue.

GET ALL THE FACTS. Analyze your information to gain as much understanding as possible about the entire situation and its real cause. You may not be able to identify or define the problem completely until you discover these basic issues. Get everyone's version of the incident, or their ideas concerning why the situation exists. Remember that emotions may influence what each person *thinks* she saw or heard. Continue to ask yourself, "Why did this happen?" as well as "What happened?"

Don't jump to a hasty conclusion. Things are not always what they appear to be at first glance. At this point it is important that you keep your thinking as objective as possible. Don't discard an observation because you think that it is contrary to what you *feel* happened. Keep an open mind. Your emotions must be controlled if you are to use the steps of problem-solving effectively. Think of yourself as a detective who considers every clue important to the case being solved.

When you have collected all the available information, sort out that which is essential to your understanding of the problem. Consider each fact by itself, then consider it in relation to the other information you have at hand. Several people may make statements which conflict; therefore, you will need to determine which is most pertinent to the situation you are considering. By this process, you are actually defining the problem. Now you are ready to go on to the next step.

DEVELOP A SOLUTION. The facts that you have collected should indicate the basic issues in this problem. You must remedy these circumstances if you are to eliminate the situation you first identified as the problem. Ask yourself, "How can I meet this situation? What are the possible results if I handle it in this way?" There are always a number of ways to solve any problem.

You may need to obtain help either from reference reading or from personal interviews. Find out what suggestions others can give. After due consideration, select the suggestion that seems to fit best in your situation.

TAKE ACTION. Do it now! Don't procrastinate! Decide how to

put your solution into effect then start working. Remember that communicating *what, why,* and *how* is important in gaining the cooperation of your team. Give everyone a chance to become acquainted with the revised way of doing things. As you talk, stress the advantages of the new method. It is human nature to resist change, but if your team members realize how they will benefit, they will be more ready to try.

EVALUATE THE RESULTS. After a trial period, determine your progress. You may not have gained all that you had hoped for, but you should be able to note some improvement. Sometimes a few minor revisions are all that is necessary to make your original plan more effective. Occasionally you may find that your selected method of solving the problem will not work at all. As a leader you cannot afford to scrap the entire project by simple shrugging your shoulders and saying that nothing can be done. Select an alternate solution and work with that for a time; eventually, you will find one that works for you. The important thing is your desire to find a workable solution. You cannot afford to become discouraged; you must continue to have self-confidence and maintain a positive attitude. There is a poem that states in part:

> Success begins with a fellow's will
> It is all in the state of mind.*

That philosophy is very important for a leader in any walk of life.

By using these five steps, you will find that you can handle *any* problem either in a directive or in a creative way. In some problems you will need to gather all the facts, do all the thinking, select what you believe to be the best solution, and inform your team of the necessary change. By doing this, you are handling the situation in a directive manner. On the other hand, you may help your team to recognize the existence of a problem, and then, with their help, develop a plan of action either through discussions with individual team members or with the team as a whole. In this way, you are solving the problem creatively. Often the cooperation of the group is strengthened when the members themselves are allowed to decide on ways of eliminating the circumstances causing the problem.

Illustration in Problem-solving. Imagine that you are having difficulty in getting your team members to report to you about their patients. You feel their failure to report is the problem; however, if you ask yourself *why,* you may find that there are underlying

---

*From *The Man Who Thinks He Can.* Anon.

HOW TO ORGANIZE YOUR WORK 61

causes, which are the real issues in this situation. Unless you discover these causes, you will never completely gain your team's cooperation in giving the desired reports. Therefore you need to do some investigating.

In this situation, you may work either directively or creatively. In either case, you must search for the answers to the questions, "Does a problem exist?" and "If one exists, what is causing it?" In team nursing, in order to insure patient-centered care, the team members, as well as their leader, must be kept informed concerning the progress of their patients. Therefore, you are justified in considering your difficulty in obtaining adequate reports to be a problem. From your personal observation, together with the information given by others, suppose you discover the following facts:

1. Team members do not always receive enough information about their patients.
2. Some team leaders expect to be told only about work that is not finished and nothing personal about the patients.
3. The team leader is not always available to receive this information from her team members.
4. Some team members do not know that a report to the team leader is required of them.
5. Some team members, especially nurses' aides and younger nursing students, do not realize what observations are important and should be reported to their team leader.

As you analyze these facts and try to understand the entire situation, you realize that a number of underlying issues exist, which are the cause of the situation first identified as the problem. You also realize that perhaps additional problems are present that you did not recognize in the beginning. In the first place, inconsistencies seem to be present in the methods used to obtain reports from the team members. Also it appears that they do not have a good example to follow. Furthermore, their lack of knowledge predisposes both to their failure to observe well and to their neglect to relay important information, even though they have obtained it.

After due consideration, suppose you decide to define your problem in this way—because the team members do not always receive a detailed report, they in turn fail to recognize the importance of relaying information. Now ask for suggestions for solving this problem. Perhaps you have some of your own, or you may be able to obtain some ideas from other team leaders who have encountered the same situation. Professional journals often contain articles with helpful suggestions for meeting the problems you may encounter in the various aspects of your work.

It is possible that you may obtain the following suggestions:
1. Ask the head nurse to inform the team members to tell their team leader what they have observed about the patients.
2. Discuss the importance of reporting with your team. Include the information you expect their report to contain and help them realize why it is important that you get their report by a certain time.
3. Give a complete report to every team member every day before she begins her work.
4. Always be available to receive reports.
5. Get a report every day even if you have to look up each team member to get it.
6. Continue to teach your team what to observe in various kinds of diseases, and why such observations are important.

Now select the solution or solutions you feel will work best in your situation. Remember to thank and praise each person when she reports to you. Indicate how much her information will help the patient, the doctor and the rest of the team, as they plan the care of the patient. Some may forget occasionally, but give them time and plenty of encouragement. Soon they will learn the value of a good report and if, in addition, you continue to instruct your team in what to watch for in their patients, you will find the quality of the reports improving also.

In a situation similar to the one used in this illustration, it is entirely inadequate simply to tell the workers that they are required to report. Such a method is extremely dictatorial and will only stimulate resentment toward you and your demands. Lack of understanding is a common reason for failure to follow procedure. You can win their cooperation more quickly by helping them to increase their understanding. Remember that a leader must go ahead and guide; she can never get behind and push.

This is a rather lengthy explanation, and makes it appear that problem-solving is time-consuming. At first, you may find that following through the various steps will take time; however, as you encounter and solve different problems, you will find that it will take less and less time to develop a workable solution because you have more experience and information to guide you.

How To Organize Your Own Work. One word of caution must be given concerning organization. Nursing care, if it is to be good, must meet all the needs of the patient—physical, emotional,

HOW TO ORGANIZE YOUR WORK

spiritual, therapeutic, and social. There is great danger that a work-plan will become so well organized that it consists only of therapeutic and physical care given on a functional basis. You must always keep in mind all the aspects of nursing care needed by the patient. In other words, refer to the entire care plan when you are organizing your work for the day. The need to find out what is troubling Mr. Smith or to give Mrs. Jones a little extra TLC (tender loving care) is something difficult to assign, yet, if the patient is to receive good nursing care, the meeting of these and other needs must be planned for.

Basically, work organization is a problem of establishing priorities, that is, determining what care is most important to each patient's welfare and arranging team activities so that each patient will receive the care he needs when he should have it. Skill in planning and organizing usually increases with experience, but you must try to improve from day to day. No one can make a set form for you to follow, but there are certain factors that, if you consider them carefully, will help you to organize your work more efficiently.

Answer these six questions as you organize your work—what? why? when? how? where? who? Every work plan should show the answers to these questions if every phase of work is to be completed. Try to ask specific questions and to formulate specific answers.

The questions *what* and *why* should be considered at the same time because they will help you to determine what care is most important to the patient's welfare. Which is more important, your spending a few minutes encouraging and showing Mrs. Jones how to move around more by herself or assigning someone to turn her at stated intervals? Should you be more concerned with giving the patient a bath and fresh linen or with helping him to understand what is happening to him and how he can help in his own recovery? As team leader you must answer the questions *what* and *why* in order to determine nursing priorities.

Answering the *what* questions will also give you a panoramic view of all the work and nursing care that your team must complete. What ward routines must be done today? What equipment and supplies are needed?

Answering the *why* questions will indicate the order in which various aspects of care should be given. Some care may need to be completed before other care can be given to the patient. If you are short of staff for the amount of work to be done (and who isn't these days?), you will find this a very important question. Consider each nursing operation, each aspect of nursing care to decide if it is really necessary. Is it necessary to give a complete bath to every patient every day? Do all baths need to be given in the morning? Must q.i.d. medications be started at 8 o'clock in the morning?

Answering the question *when* will also help in arranging the order in which care should be given, or in determining what duties may be combined to save time and steps. Plan to give the patient as much of his care as possible at one time. Conversations, carried on during the bath or a treatment, should contain more than incidental pleasantries; they should be made worth while by meeting some need of the patient.

You will need to estimate the length of time each aspect of care will take in order to avoid conflicts in the work of the various team members. For example, if you are to start an intravenous feeding after a patient has been given her morning care, you will need to know how long the worker, assigned to give that care, will need to complete it. Furthermore, answering these questions will help you have all equipment available when it is needed.

To answer the question *how*, you may need to refer to the hospital policy book, the procedure manual, and the patient's care plan, or you may want to do some research on your own. Is one method of arranging duties better than another? Can you save a few steps by rearranging the equipment or by changing the method of handling supplies? For instance, instead of walking back and forth between linen closet and the patients' rooms, perhaps you can devise a linen cart. Soiled linen could be placed in a linen hamper, which the worker moves with her, rather than disposing of the linen down a distant laundry chute after the care of each patient. Try to obtain all supplies and equipment at one time. Saving steps and eliminating unnecessary motions are a saving of time and energy, which can be used to give more nursing care. Time and motion studies are basically problem solving in nature. A nurse must be ready to change her work methods, always looking for more efficient ways to decrease the quantity of work motions, and, at the same time, improving the quality of nursing care.

You must also answer the question *where*. The geographical location of care to be given will definitely affect the time necessary to complete it. The more centralized you can make a certain number of duties, the easier it will be for the worker.

Very important in team nursing is the answer to the question *who*. Can this duty be delegated to one of the team members? If so, who is best qualified to give this part of the patient's care? There are some responsibilities you cannot delegate; on the other hand, you should not think that you must give all the care. Choosing the right person for the job is important, because you must consider not only the patient and his needs, but also the worker and her needs. Part of your responsibility as team leader is to help each of

HOW TO ORGANIZE YOUR WORK

your team members increase her understanding and skill in giving nursing care. Team members must be given the opportunity to acquire these new skills. The principles involved in making assignments to your team members will be discussed in more detail.

If difficulties arise as you plan your work, apply the rules for solving problems. You should also attempt to prevent difficult situations from occurring.

FORESEE POSSIBLE EMERGENCIES AND PLAN ACCORDINGLY. Since planning means thinking ahead, you must include more than the organization of duties that you know must be completed. From your experience as a nurse, you know that emergencies arise constantly no matter how well-organized the hospital ward may be. For example, a patient suddenly becomes critically ill; or a new patient is admitted who requires your constant attention. Try to leave yourself and your team some loopholes, so that these expected emergencies can be taken care of with a minimum amount of confusion and rearrangement of your initial plan. For example, you may have assigned extra duties that, if an emergency arises, can be omitted for that day or done at a different time. Should it become necessary, make the adjustments in the assignments. If the emergency does not develop, you have already planned how to use the time profitably by completing this additional work. If you are reasonably sure that a number of patients will be admitted, adjust the current workload of one individual and assign her to care for the new patients.

PUT YOUR PLAN IN WRITING. This plan must include more than patient assignments and the nursing care to be given by your team, although these items will occupy a major portion. Do not trust yourself to remember all the details; write them down for future reference. Again, a set form cannot be given to fit your situation. You will need to work out your own; however, you will probably want to include, in addition to the patient care assignments, the following:

1. A list of routine ward duties to be done, e.g., clean dressing cart, check all dresser drawers for extra blankets.
2. Reminders to yourself concerning duties that require your special attention, e.g., getting special equipment ready for a doctor, observing and teaching your team members, teaching a particular patient.
3. Notations concerning help in giving bedside nursing care needed by any of your team members.
4. Questions or observations that you want to bring to the attention of the head nurse or doctor.
5. Incidental duties needing your attention, e.g., meetings to attend.

HOW TO PREPARE YOUR TEAM

Cultivating Team Spirit. Whether you are working in an area where team nursing has been practiced for some time or are in the process of instituting the team plan, proper preparation of all personnel is necessary if team spirit is to develop. The spirit of cooperation within the team necessary for effective group action, begins with your own belief in the philosophy of team nursing and with your attitudes toward your work and toward your team members as individuals. You must be enthusiastic about this method of planning nursing care, for, if you are not, your own feelings of resentment and defeat will be transmitted to your team, and you will never win their full cooperation. You must recognize that each person has something worthwhile to contribute to the welfare of the patient, and, in addition, you must be able to communicate to each team member your appreciation of her capabilities. You must have a sincere desire to be a leader, not for the glory of the title or the position, but for the satisfaction you obtain from working with and helping people.

The focal point in cultivating team spirit is having a common goal — in this case, the giving of good nursing care. In all that you and your team do, this thought must be emphasized — together, the team can give better nursing care than a number of people working independently.

All members of the team must understand the principles upon which the team plan is founded and the way in which it functions. They must understand the ways of coordinating all activities of the individual members of the team to provide total nursing care for the patient. They must understand the reasons for, and the methods of using, the conference and the nursing care plan for planning and giving patient care. This information should be explained to them before team nursing is started. They should be allowed to ask questions and to discuss how the team plan would affect them and their work. Even after the team plan is instituted, this instruction should be continued, especially as new employees join the group. The team leader is the one who must reinforce this instruction by giving additional explanations, but she will generate the best enthusiasm and cooperation by her own example.

You cannot set yourself apart from your team. Telling them to work together will never be so effective as working with them yourself. Your actions must demonstrate the idea of *our* work together, rather than *your* work and *my* work.

You cannot stop at the end of the preliminary period of preparation if your group is to develop into a team, cemented together by a spirit of cooperation and a desire to achieve the common goal.

Team spirit must be continually nurtured and encouraged to grow. Each person has the basic need for approval. She wants to do that which will satisfy this need, but in order to do so, she must know what she is to do and how to do it. Communication is important in any cooperative effort. Your ability to put your ideas across and to receive ideas from others is essential to the mutual understanding that must precede effective team work. You must help each person to gain a clear understanding of what she is to do and how her work is important to the patient. Show confidence in her ability to do her work, then do not forget to praise her for work well-done, or to criticize constructively and fairly when she should be better.

Not only must the individual be given recognition and help, but also the team as a whole. Emphasize that each person as a member of the team shares in the responsibility for giving good patient care, and that, when the patient is satisfied, the entire team, not one individual alone, shares in the credit.

Orientation Must Precede Assignment of Duties. Webster defines the word *orient* as "to set right by adjusting to facts or principles; to put into correct position or relation, to acquaint with the existing situation." Any orientation must include information concerning not only the physical set-up of the station and the hospital, but also what the person's specific duties and responsibilities are.

The method of presentation, as well as the information included, will vary according to the aim of the orientation and the needs of the individual. Probably you will not have to orient a new employee to the ward since the head nurse usually assumes this responsibility herself; however, orientation should be continued for several days until the person becomes acquainted with the ward situation in which she is to work. Remember the individual needs to feel secure in what she is doing. The more inexperienced she is, the more she feels the need for this security. If she does not know how to obtain supplies or information, or what work standards must be met, her feeling of insecurity is increased and, as a result, she may be unable to do her work satisfactorily or to receive personal satisfaction from her work. A person can rarely remember all the information given during the planned orientation program; therefore, you must continue to give her help by repeating and adding to the information whenever she needs it.

The new employee is not the only one who needs orientation. When a worker returns from a holiday or vacation, or after her regular days off, she will need to be brought up-to-date on new patients and any changes in policy or hospital routines that have been made while she was away. Again the amount of information and the method of giving it will vary according to the experience of the person and the responsibilities she must assume.

In any orientation, but especially that of a new employee, whenever you discover an area in which a team member needs more understanding, you should make plans for teaching her. Perhaps she has had several years' experience in another hospital. Remember that procedures and terminology differ from place to place. For example, the early postoperative exercises may be described in one hospital as turn, cough, and hyperventilate; in another they may be abbreviated to T, C, and H. Another place may use the term, *stir-ups*, to describe the same procedure. Make sure that she is familiar with the terms commonly used on your ward. Perhaps you mention that the postoperative bed, which she is assigned to make, will need the covers fanfolded to the left side. Noting her puzzled expression, you discover that she is used to folding the covers to the foot of the bed. These may seem to be such little things to one who is familiar with them, but to a stranger they become obstacles hindering the satisfactory performance of her work. Helping her to become acquainted with the existing situation will result in a more satisfied and happier person on your team, one who will look up to you and think of you as a wonderful team leader.

Encourage all team members to ask questions. These may indicate to you those areas in which additional information is needed by the group. As you observe your team in action, other areas may show up. From time to time you may need to go over various procedures and routines with your team as a whole. New policies and procedures always mean that you must orient your team to these changes.

HOW TO GIVE A GOOD PATIENT REPORT

A report is one form of orientation, because its purpose is to impart information about the existing situation; therefore, it is used to prepare the personnel for their day's work. Complete, concise reports are vital to good management and administration. No team can function efficiently without this method of communication. Every team member, whether she is a graduate nurse or a nurses' aide, should have some knowledge of the patient's condition, including his problems and suggested methods for helping him, as well as of his treatment and progress. A report will give each person this information quickly.

You will have occasion to use many kinds of reports; however, at this time the emphasis will be on the patient condition report. This report is given before the team members start their work for the day and is not the nursing care conference. As team leader, any information about your patients is important to you and to each of your team members. You must receive a report from the previous team leaders, and you must pass on that information to your team. They, in turn, should report to you their observations, as well as their progress in caring for the patients. Their information, combined with your own observations, will then need to be relayed back to the head nurse and to the oncoming team leaders. This constant exchange of information is essential to make your leadership effective, and to provide good patient care.

A well-informed team will be more cooperative and unified team. In order to give adequate nursing care, everyone in the group must receive a report about her patients. Here are some suggestions designed to make your team reports more complete and helpful.

Every Report Must Be Given Promptly. Other duties can be taken care of later, or someone can be assigned to care for an emergency if one exists. A delay in giving the report contributes to confusion, which in turn leads to further delay and to errors in giving necessary nursing care. Changes in a patient's condition may alter the methods of giving his care. Each person must be informed of these changes to insure safe nursing care for the patient. Most errors can be traced to a breakdown in communication, frequently in the giving, or not giving, of a report. Since, as team leader, you are responsible for all nursing care given by your team, you are also responsible for giving them the necessary information so that they can perform their duties properly. Organized leadership demands that a thorough, concise report be given promptly at the scheduled time.

Always Call Each Patient by Name. Nothing destroys the individuality of a person as quickly as speaking of him as "the appy in room 4204, bed 2." He ceases to be a real person and becomes instead a disease and a bed number. Calling the patient by name not only identifies the exact person about whom you are speaking, but also helps your team to think of him as an individual. Of course, you will need to include other information such as room number, doctor's name and patient's diagnosis, but these are important only because you have first identified as a real person the patient to whom they belong.

Always Use the Entire Patient Care Plan as a Guide in Giving a Complete Picture of Your Patient. This plan includes the therapeutic treatment of medical problems prescribed by the doctor and delegated to the nurse. It also includes the treatment of nursing problems as identified by you and your team. Information from both areas is necessary if the patient is to receive total care. The report should also include information concerning what has been done for the patient and how he responded, as well as what should be done and how to do it. Be sure to call the attention of your group to any changes that have occurred in the patient's condition. Report any deviation from routine methods in carrying out the physician's orders or the nursing care, e.g., specific observations to be made, topics of conversation to be avoided, or the specific time when certain care is to be given.

Keep the Report on a Professional Level. Avoid gossiping or saying derogatory things about any patient. Sometimes the question arises concerning how much information to include in the report to the team members or in the discussions during the team conferences. Perhaps the best way to decide this question is to determine if the information will help the workers to understand the patient and his illness, thereby enabling them to give better nursing care. If the answer is *yes*, give them the information. Remember that the nurses' aide and the practical nurse are the ones who spend the most time with the patient; consequently, the patient may tell them more of his personal problems than we realize. It is important that your team members understand what the patient can and cannot do and why, so that everyone can give safe nursing care and correct information to the patient. They need to recognize, although they may not understand, the relationship between the patient's disease and his behavior. For instance, they would be more sympathetic toward the patient who has suffered a stroke if they recognize that his irritability may be a symptom, or the result, of his physical condition. Or they will be better prepared to care for the patient with multiple sclerosis if they know beforehand that the fact that this patient laughs one minute and cries the next is a manifestation of the disease and is not related to anything they have said or done.

The following incident also emphasizes the need for complete explanation of the patient's treatment. An order for "No Smoking" was left for a patient who was to have lung surgery; however, he continually begged everyone for just one cigarette. Finally, a nurses' aide, feeling sorry for him, gave him one, saying, "This little bit can't hurt you." Had the team leader explained the reason for this order and indicated what information to give to the patient, all of the team members would have had a better understanding of this patient and would have been better prepared to meet his demands.

Of course, the giving of a good report takes time; however, a good report combined with a well-explained assignment will save you time later and will help to insure safer and better patient care. Foreseeing the questions your team may want answered, and giving them the necessary explanations before they start their work, will result in fewer interruptions, allowing you more time to carry out your own duties and give additional help to your team. On the other hand, your team will be able to go ahead with a greater feeling of confidence because they know what they should do and how to do it.

Another common problem involves the reporting to persons who come in at odd hours. If your head nurse has one or more such individuals assigned to your team, some provision must be made so that they will obtain all the information they need to carry out their assignments safely and without unnecessary delay. It must be stressed that giving them an assignment sheet on which is indicated the work they are to do is not the same as a report, and, if such a method is followed, you have no right to expect the individual to do her best.

As a rule, the team report and assignments are given simultaneously. To save time some hospitals have all team members attend the patient report given by the previous shift; then each group meets separately to receive additional information about individual assignments.

HOW TO MAKE A GOOD ASSIGNMENT

A good report is the beginning of a good assignment. Assignments in team nursing should include all the duties necessary for the smooth functioning of the ward, as well as the nursing care of the patients assigned to the team by the head nurse. Individual assignments should not be based on the functional method of assigning various duties to different people. If the team is to work together on a level above that of giving functional care, they must be concerned with more than just getting the work done. Your philosophy as team leader is important in this respect for you will practice what you believe. The work itself should never be considered more important than the patient or the worker. When emphasis is on the work alone, both the quality and the quanity of work decline.

You must coordinate the activities of your team in order to provide patient-centered care. In nursing there are some areas which cannot be assigned, or at least are difficult to assign, on a functional basis; consequently, they are often omitted when that method of assignment is used. For example how can you assign one person to give encouragement to the patient who is afraid or depressed, or to give that personal touch, sometimes called tender loving care, or to allow a patient to talk about his troubles? As team leader you are the only one who can insure that all needs of the patient are met. This can be done only if everyone on your team knows what should be done for each patient and plans together how to do it.

Common Mistakes Made in Giving Directions. If you and your team are to accomplish anything, everyone must know and understand what she is to do. Here are several reasons why your directions are sometimes not carried out as you intended.

The most common mistakes are: speaking indistinctly, talking too fast, or using words not understood by the worker. When you are in a hurry, do you slur your words, or leave out words, or use abbreviations for technical terms? Do you take for granted that the person will understand what you mean? One team leader directed a nurses' aide to, "Check Mrs. Jones for discharge." What she meant was "for drainage"; however, the aide thought she meant to check Mrs. Jones "to go home." The rules for effective communications must be constantly observed when giving directions.

Another common mistake is giving directions in a disorganized or haphazard fashion. It is extremely difficult to remember what to do if the leader goes back several times to include some information or direction she forgot to put in its proper place. Make sure that you know what you want the person to do and how you want her to do it, then tell her step by step. Don't rush through it; give yourself, as well as the other person, time to think about what you are saying.

Giving too many directions at one time is confusing to the person who must follow them. This is especially true if the directions are given verbally and without regard to logical order. You must consider the experience of the individual when giving her directions. The less experience she has, the simpler you must make your orders. If there are many things to do, the directions must be placed in writing to serve as a reminder and to safeguard against any omission.

Poor grammar may result in misunderstanding. The placement of words in a sentence gives meaning by indicating relationship. When placement is wrong, the exact meaning is lost. Faulty pronouns of reference are especially likely to result in such misunderstanding.

The pronouns *it, this, that, those, them* must be used carefully. For example, "Put *it* on *that* shelf over there" could be very confusing if the person did not know what *it, that shelf,* and *over there* referred to specifically. For clarity, use the exact word rather than a pronoun, or use each pronoun so that there is no question concerning its reference.

One of the biggest mistakes is assuming that your directions are understood. What seems very simple to you may appear very difficult to someone else. It is always dangerous to assume that any individual understood what you said just because you told her once. The interpretation of an idea is always based upon the listener's past learning and experience. Always make sure that each member understands exactly what she is to do and when and how to do it; for example, you may ask her to repeat your directions or you may ask her questions about how she is going to complete her assignment.

Making Individual Assignments. When making out the assignments for your team members, you must always consider both the patient and worker. Nor can the needs of the patient always be considered before the needs of the person who is to care for him. In order to do her best, each team member must feel satisfied with her job. Here are a few suggestions designed to help you in making assignments to your individual team members.

HAVE A THOROUGH KNOWLEDGE OF YOUR JOB. This is one quality team members consider to be very important. They want the person leading them to be capable of giving them intelligent help and guidance. This means that you must know what nursing care is needed by your patients and the best way to give it. You must

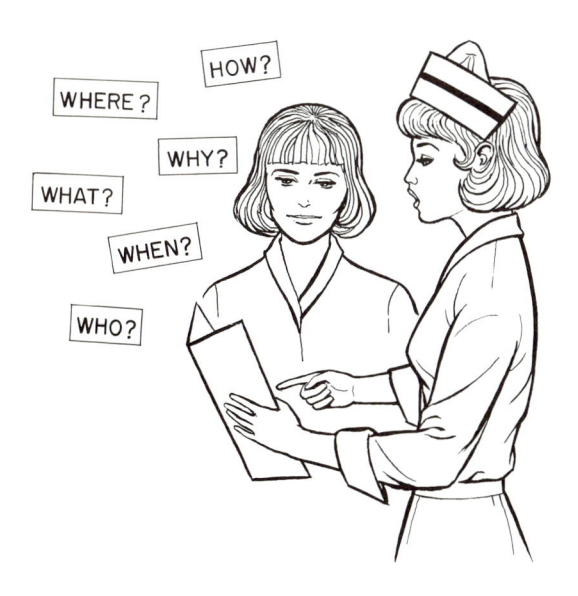

Figure 3. *Directions must be complete.*

know where and how to obtain the necessary supplies, equipment, and information. You must be aware of the other duties that should be completed and recognize their relationship to the functioning of the ward as a whole. You need an over-all plan for your team and a more specific plan for your own work. You must be able to communicate effectively and to maintain good human relationships.

CONSIDER EACH WORKER AS AN INDIVIDUAL. Making out assignments is more than dividing the total number of patients by the total number of people available on your team, thereby assigning everyone the same number of patients to care for. An assignment, if it is to provide for good nursing care, cannot be based on number of patients only, nor is an equal division of work always fair if number of duties alone is considered. To make out a good assignment you should consider each worker as an individual and make her assignment based on these factors: it should be related to her previous experience; it should provide for new learning experiences or for the reinforcement of skills recently learned; it should be within her ability to complete; it should be interesting; it should provide a sense of satisfaction.

New responsibilities are always challenging and stimulating. Of course, you must make certain that each person knows how to do the work assigned to her, or, if not, plan to teach her as she works. In addition, you must follow hospital policies in assigning specific duties to the proper person.

An assignment must be fair, yet within the ability of the worker to complete it. It should be stimulating enough to make her want to learn more and to do her best. On any hospital ward there are a number of routine, somewhat boring, tasks that must be done if the ward is to run smoothly. Don't give all these tasks to one person. Spread them out or combine them with new or more interesting duties. It is very unwise to take advantage of the willing worker or to show favoritism in any way. Whenever possible, rotate duties so that everyone becomes acquainted with all the patients and has a chance to learn all of the ward routines they are capable of doing.

When assigning the number of patients to be cared for by any one individual, you must consider the amount of care each patient needs and the time necessary to complete that care. You must also take into account the rate of speed with which the individual performs her work, although you cannot penalize the rest of the team by giving one member a smaller assignment because she is a slow worker. Rather you should try to determine why she is unable to complete a usual assignment in an average length of time, then help her to do better.

PROVIDE FOR INDIVIDUALIZED NURSING CARE FOR EACH PATIENT. Use the care plan for meeting nursing problems, along

HOW TO ORGANIZE YOUR WORK

with the plan for treatments and medications. You would never think of planning your work without first knowing what treatments or medications are ordered for your patients. In like manner, you, and each of your team members, should know what techniques have been suggested to solve the individual problems of each patient, then plan to use them.

As you assign the various patients or certain aspects of their care to your team members, you need to rely on your preliminary planning in which you have already determined what, when, where, how, and who. Choosing the person who is best equipped to give the patient the kind of care he needs is no small task, nor one that should be thought of lightly. Consider the skills necessary to give him good care, then choose the proper person carefully. In addition the rapport, built up between patient and team member, is important to the welfare of both.

FIX RESPONSIBILITY FOR ALL DUTIES CLEARLY WITH NO OVERLAPPING. Again you need to refer to your own work plan to insure that all duties have been assigned to someone; however, two people should never be assigned to do the same thing, for there is danger that each will rely upon the other to perform the entire task with the result that neither does it. A broad assignment, such as cleaning the utility room, unless it is to be done by one person, can be improved by breaking it into its separate parts, then assigning each individual certain duties.

For the same reason, two people should not be assigned to care for the same patient. If certain parts of care for this patient must be done by two people, be very specific about what each is to do. If an aide can give most of the care, perhaps a nursing student or yourself can be assigned to "help" with those specific aspects of care that she cannot perform or that require more than one person. Assigning a nurse to give "medications and treatments" to those patients who receive part of their care from nurses' aides can be confusing when the aides are able to give some of the treatments but not all of them. Furthermore, there is danger that this kind of assignment may degenerate into a functional method of doing the work. When you make your assignments definite and clear-cut, you are more likely to have them completed properly. In addition, it is easier for you to determine if they have been completed, and, if not, who is responsible for failing to do so.

ARRANGE THE VARIOUS PARTS OF THE ASSIGNMENT IN LOGICAL ORDER AND EXPLAIN CLEARLY AND CONCISELY. Depending upon the experience of the worker, you may need to indicate the best time to perform the various duties assigned to her. If a certain part of a patient's care must be completed in order to allow someone else time to do something more for that patient, you must so indicate in the assignment and call the worker's attention to it as you go over the assignment with her. Give additional explanation about terms and methods of performance whenever there is some question about whether or not the worker understands what she is to do or how to do it.

PUT ASSIGNMENTS IN WRITING TO SERVE AS A GUIDE WHILE WORKING AND TO INSURE THAT NO PART IS OMITTED. Sometimes additional directions may need to be included. This is especially true for patient assignment and the special aspects of nursing care, but it may also be necessary for ward routines, such as cleaning the dressing cart or checking the linen room. Some team leaders note these special directions on the individual assignment sheets as they make them out. Others train their team members to make their own notations as they listen to the report and the explanation about their duties.

Incidental orders or directions, given after the main assignment has been explained, may need to be put in writing, depending upon their importance. Telling an aide to take a glassfull of fresh water to a patient is one thing, but telling her to give an enema, which has just been ordered by the doctor, is another. The first need not be written, the second should be, especially if the aide is unable to give the enema immediately.

MAKE CERTAIN THAT EVERYONE UNDERSTANDS HER ASSIGNMENT. If you have prepared the assignment carefully and explained it thoroughly, your team members should know what they are expected to do. However, never assume that they understand what you have told them. Repeat if necessary. Encourage questions. Foresee possible questions and answer them as you go along.

ANTICIPATE AND, AS MUCH AS POSSIBLE, PROVIDE FOR EMERGENCY SITUATIONS AND SPECIAL NURSING ACTIVITIES. A new surgical patient may start to bleed. A doctor may wish to do a lengthy examination. The x-ray department will call for a patient earlier than expected. Even the best laid plans cannot always be completed according to the original schedule. Try to prepare your team for possible emergencies. Remember that planning means looking ahead. Every plan should be flexible enough to allow for changes if the need arises.

OBSERVE AND CHECK THE PERFORMANCE OF EACH TEAM MEMBER. No assignment is complete until you are satisfied that it has been performed as you intended. You should not, however, nag or stand over a person to insure adequate performance. Indicating your confidence in your team's ability to do good work will usually encourage each one to do her best. On the other hand, your own observations are necessary, along with a report from each team member about her patients and her work, if you are to obtain a complete picture of the care each patient received. There are many methods of observation which you may choose. Some of these will be discussed in the following chapter.

Your Manner in Giving Directions Is Important. As a team leader, you must learn how to work and get along with people. The manner in which you give directions and explain assignments will indicate to your team your attitude about them as individuals. Always keep in mind that you are working *with* them, that they are never working *for* you. The degree to which your leadership is creative, and the situation itself, will determine to a great extent the manner in which you give directions.

THERE ARE TIMES WHEN YOU WILL NEED TO GIVE A DIRECT ORDER OR COMMAND. In case of emergency or danger, when time is important, you are the only one who has the necessary knowledge; therefore, you tell each person just what to do. Sometimes in order to control certain types of individuals, e.g., the one who is lazy or indifferent, or who refuses to follow accepted procedures, you will find that the direct approach is more effective than any other.

YOU MAY OCCASIONALLY USE AN IMPLIED DIRECTION. When your team has learned to work together efficiently and has gained more experience, you can sometimes suggest the action that you want taken. For example, you enter a patient's room while his care is being given and find it somewhat cooler than you believe is safe for the patient. You may say, "It seems rather chilly in here." The experienced worker will get the hint. You may also use this approach to stimulate a person to develop more initiative.

YOU MAY WANT TO CALL FOR VOLUNTEERS. This is a valuable method when a disagreeable job needs to be done, or when extra work needs to be done. Do not allow the group to depend upon one individual's volunteering all the time. Also you will help strengthen team spirit if you offer to help whoever volunteers.

THE MOST COMMON METHOD OF GIVING DIRECTIONS IS BY MAKING THEM IN THE FORM OF A REQUEST. There are many different ways for wording a direction in this manner, for instance, "Will you . . . ?" or "Let's . . ." or "How about . . . ?" This method stimulates cooperation and helps get more work done. It works well with the person who is extremely "touchy" or with one who is your equal in rank. It will also work with the person who is interested in her job, or with the individual who is older than you are and may, therefore, dislike taking orders from you.

Your own preparation, as well as that of your team, is important in keeping the work of the team moving ahead smoothly. It is during this time that you either win or lose their cooperation and confidence for the day. Needless to say, how they feel toward you will be reflected in the quality of nursing care they give. You must be able to inspire their confidence in you as a leader by displaying self-confidence but not conceit, by being firm but not intolerant, by formulating plans that are well-organized but not rigid, by considering the needs of the individual, yet not forgetting the welfare of the group.

HOW TO KEEP ORGANIZED

Remember that planning is a continuous process. Rarely will you be able to complete your original plan without change. If a rearrangement of duties becomes necessary, you need to evaluate the situation, changing as little as possible, in order to minimize confusion and chance of error.

Carry Your Work Plan with You at All Times. Do not trust your memory. Review your plan periodically to insure that nothing is forgotten. Always refer to it before starting each part of your assignment. Make notes on the information that needs to be recorded on the patient's chart or relayed to the head nurse. Jot down ideas for your closer consideration about improving the efficiency of your team.

Help Your Team To Keep Organized. Although you are responsible for planning and directing the work being done by your team, you must also help each person to develop her ability to plan her own work. If she is to use her time to the best advantage, she must be able to organize her duties.

GIVE EACH PERSON TIME AND OPPORTUNITY TO PLAN HER WORK. In order to plan what she is to do, a worker must be able to answer the same six questions—what, why, when, how, where, and who. However, she will not need to answer them as completely as you did. You must give a complete patient report to your team. In addition, you will need to give additional explantion concerning the individual assignments. This is especially important when several people are concerned with different aspects of care for the same patient. As a rule, most team members are able to plan the sequence of their work while you give the report and explain their assignments. You may need to give additional help and suggestions concerning possible arrangement of duties to the inexperienced worker or to one who has been having difficulties in completing her usual assignment. Remember your example of good organization will help her in planning her own work.

If you have a nursing student on your team, she should be expected, depending upon the amount of clinical experience she has had, to develop a well-organized plan and to carry out that plan satisfactorily. As the duties increase in number and the responsibilities become more demanding, some students experience difficulty in determining the relative importance of the many tasks to which they have been assigned, and they do not know where to begin. Although this is a normal situation in the process of learning, it can be quite frustrating to the student unless she is able to obtain the necessary help. You are as much responsible for the personal growth of the nursing student as you are for any other member of your team; however, the explanations you give to her should be more complete than those you give to a nurses' aide. The ability to formulate workable plans can come only through practice; therefore, the student must be given the opportunity to plan her work and be allowed sufficient time to execute it. Furthermore, she must be helped to evaluate the effectiveness of her plan and to realize how to do better next time.

HAVE ALL NECESSARY SUPPLIES AND EQUIPMENT AVAILABLE. Having planned how she is going to do her work, the individual is anxious to begin. Nothing is more frustrating and time-consuming than looking for supplies someone has misplaced or forgotten to order. You are responsible for having all necessary equipment and supplies available when they are needed. If you wish, you may assign this duty to one of your team before the rest of the day's work is begun. It is wise, however, to use a written list as a guide so that nothing will be omitted.

EXCEPT IN CASE OF AN EMERGENCY, AVOID INTERRUPTING YOUR TEAM WHILE THEY ARE WORKING. A well-planned day should eliminate many of the reasons for taking a person away from her work to run errands or to begin some new task. Try to anticipate changes that may occur in the treatment of your patients, and forewarn your team members to expect these changes and plan accordingly. When a person is interrupted in her work, she loses not only the time needed to perform the new assignment but also the time used to pick up where she left off. Frequent interruptions are one reason why many team members are unable to complete their work on time.

ENCOURAGE AND HELP EACH TEAM MEMBER TO IMPROVE HER WORK HABITS. The person must recognize those areas in which her planning was weak or the reasons why she was unable to complete her work. Help her to evaluate her plan. Suggest changes that may improve it. Help her to realize whether or not she is organized while she works. Does she remember to take all the supplies she needs when she first goes to her patient's room, or does she make several trips to pick up items she forgot? Does she save time by combining several aspects of care? If not, you will need to help her to think ahead more efficiently. Perhaps she moves slowly; you will need to analyze whether this is a personal characteristic or whether a health problem exists. Sometimes individuals are unable to complete their work on time, not because they are slow workers, but because they waste time. Perhaps they procrastinate in starting their work, or they may become sidetracked into doing some insignificant duties not directly related to the patient's care. Whatever the cause, you will need to help each one improve her habits in planning and doing her work.

Evaluate the Effectiveness of Your Planning. You should be able to decide whether you and your team have completed all the work in the day's assignment within the allotted time. Determine if your patients are satisfied with the care they received. Find out if your team members are satisfied. The information you obtain in these two areas will help to indicate the results of your plan. If certain weak areas appear, indicating that better organization could have been used, determine what was wrong with the original plan, then try to avoid these mistakes the next time.

At first this process of planning will take some time, but, with practice, you will discover how various aspects of your work fit together most efficiently. A few minutes spent in this preliminary organization will save minutes, or even hours, later in the day. In addition, much of the aimless confusion, which is a source of tension and frustration for both you and your team members, can be eliminated.

QUESTIONS ABOUT WORK ORGANIZATION

Why don't people do things the way they are supposed to? I wish I knew a good answer to this. Instead of generalizing, perhaps we should put the question in more personal terms. Why don't you do things the way you are supposed to? If you can answer this, then you will know why others fail. Of course if everyone did everything correctly, there would be no problems. We must keep in mind that no one, including ourselves, is perfect; therefore, no one, again including ourselves, will do things in the way in which they are supposed to be done every time. This does not mean, however, that we can stop trying. As professional people we must supply that incentive, for ourselves as well as for others, that will enable us to improve constantly as we work toward our goal.

Should there be one report only, for everyone, or should there be one report for the nurses and one for the team members? My personal belief is that it makes little difference if everyone receives one report or if the team leaders hear the report given by the previous shift, then relay the pertinent information to their teams.

There are arguments both pro and con. The important point is that everyone must have a patient report and receive an explanation of her assignment. I believe that as a professional group we are so concerned about the possibility of giving too much information to the nonprofessional personnel that we fail to recognize our responsibility for helping them to use correctly the information they obtain from other sources.

Should the head nurse or the team leader report to the oncoming shift? Whichever method is used, there must be good communication between head nurse and team leader. Since the head nurse has the over-all responsibility for everything that goes on in her unit, she must be kept fully informed by the team leaders, concerning their work and any difficulties they encounter. The head nurse, in turn, must relay all pertinent information to the team leaders if they are to function properly. The head nurse may wish to delegate to the team leader the responsibility for reporting on those patients cared for by her team; however, the head nurse must attend this report to insure its completeness by supplying additional information whenever necessary.

How can a registered nurse, when she works part-time and must relieve either the team leader or ancillary personnel, fit into the team? We need to consider first the definition of *part-time*. Some hospitals consider a person to be part-time if she works a full 40-hour week but will not rotate shifts or week ends. Other hospitals consider those persons to be part-time who work less than the prescribed number of hours each week or each month. Such a person may work 4 hours daily, 4 or 5 days a week, or 1 or 2 8-hour days each week.

As a general rule, the fewer the hours worked each week, or the more widely spaced those hours are within the week, the more difficult it would be, I believe, for this nurse to assume the responsibilities of team leadership. Her unfamiliarity with the patients, their needs, and their treatment would make it almost impossible for her to give more than functional care. Furthermore, she would probably have to refer the questions asked by her team to the head nurse. This practice of referring them to someone else for advice was one point criticized often by the nurses' aides in answer to their questionnaire, and may have been the reason for their comment that they liked best the team leader "who knows her job."

If, of necessity the part-time nurse must work as team leader, even though she is not acquainted with the patients, she must receive a thorough report and orientation to her patients from the head nurse. In addition, the head nurse will need to work more closely with her throughout the day, helping her to direct and supervise the work of her team. The head nurse may also have to assume the responsibility for conducting the team conference and checking the nursing care plans.

It would be much better if the part-time registered nurse, especially if she works only one or two days a week, could be assigned as a member of a team, relieving the team leader of some of her responsibilities, such as helping the team members care for those patients who are most ill. In this way the team leader will have more time for the supervision of the team as a whole.

How can assignments be made according to the aides' abilities? According to hospital policy, nurses' aides may perform certain procedures and duties. However, simply because the policy states that she can be assigned to do a certain task does not indicate her skill in performing it. If there is a very ill patient who needs skillful nursing care, you would want to assign the person who is best qualified to give this care. However, we need to consider more than just the worker's experience and dexterity. We need to give some thought to her personality, interests, physical limitations, and her ability to get along with people. We must make use of these qualities, matching them to the patients. For example, the worker who has a sunny disposition and seems to get along well with people could be assigned to the patient who is inclined to be irritable, or the patient who likes to talk could be cared for by the team member who does not find topics of conversation readily. In addition, an assignment should be made so that each person can use those abilities which she has and also have the opportunity to gain more experience.

How can team nursing be carried on when one team leader goes off duty at noon, leaving one other team leader on duty until 3 o'clock? Before the one leader leaves, she should report to the other team leader about the nursing her team has completed and what remains to be done. The two teams then become one larger team under the direction of the remaining team leader. At times, the head nurse may be the only professional nurse on duty. She then becomes the leader not only because she is head nurse and is responsible for all nursing care which her patients receive but also because as a professional nurse she must assume responsibility for directing and supervising the personnel with less knowledge than herself.

What specific assignments should the team leader give herself? What you do is determined by your personal philosophy about nursing and nursing care, by the abilities of your team members, and by hospital policy. In team nursing the team leader should do those things for the patient which others on the team cannot do because of lack of knowledge or skill or because hospital policy forbids. In other words you will need to give nursing care (not just do nursing procedures) because your team members cannot give the kind of care that your patient needs. You may be the one who should bathe and care for a critically ill patient, or work with a patient, helping him to drink more fluids, or talk with a patient who is worried about the pain in his back.

Personally, I do not feel that the team leader must give *all* the medications or do *all* the charting if there is someone else on the team who can assume responsibility for these techniques. If we allow the nurses' aide and the licensed practical nurse to give all the bedside care that a patient needs, perhaps the professional nurse is not needed after all. Rather than functioning as "medical assistants," we should concern ourselves with our primary responsibility—nursing care.

How can a team leader do her own work for the day? Whenever possible you should start your planning on the day preceding the use of the plans. You can start as soon as you know what personnel will be on your team and what patients you will be caring for. If you know these patients, you will be familiar with the care each one needs. If not, now is the time to become acquainted. Ideally, the team leader should be given the responsibility of planning the assignments for her team members; however this may be modified to meet the policies of each hospital. If you do have this responsibility, you may want to arrange the assignments on the preceding day also, although it is permissible to wait until you have visited each patient after hearing the patient report. In either case, you should give some preliminary thought to the duties to be done on the following day and how they can be organized. Much of the preliminary planning involves evaluating each patient and his needs and determining priorities in nursing techniques and care.

After you hear the patient report from the previous shift, you will need to visit each patient to evaluate his current condition for yourself. Your team members may be passing out bath supplies, taking temperatures, or doing other incidental duties during this time. You will not be able to spend much time with each patient; therefore, you should plan beforehand what you wish to observe and what information to obtain from the patient. Use this information, together with that obtained from the report, to adjust or make out the team assignments according to the needs of the patients and the abilities of your team members. Determine which patients need to receive their care first and how to correlate your care with that to be given by other departments within the hospital.

Your group should meet together to receive their report, or, if they attend the one given by the previous shift, you should meet together now to discuss the assignments and the methods of coordinating the activities of the team as a whole. Knowing how everyone will be working together encourages team spirit and the desire to participate.

As your team members carry out their duties, you do those things you had planned for yourself. In addition, you must circulate among your team members, helping with and directing the care they are giving. This is an important aspect in the leadership of your team. Give praise for good work, correct and teach when necessary, encourage the group to work together, be available and willing to answer questions and to help with the care of patients as necessary. If you have many duties of your own, finding the time to circulate in this way becomes a problem, yet it must be done if you are to lead your group. Perhaps you can delegate some of your other duties to another team member. Sometimes the problem is one of better work organization. Whatever the situation, you must plan to give this help as you go about your own duties.

Throughout the day, a continuous flow of communication is necessary between patient and team, including yourself; between you and your team members; and between the head nurse and yourself. Communication is a necessary ingredient of coordinated activity and effective team work.

Cooperative planning of nursing care occurs during the team conference under your guidance and direction. As a result, the nursing care plans are kept up-to-date, and necessary revisions are made when changes in the patient's progress are indicated by your own observations and by the reports of your team members.

Your team members should report to you immediately when they observe anything significant about the patient or when they encounter any problem in the care of the patient; however, you will need to teach them what is important, for they will not always realize what is significant and what is not. These reports cannot take the place of the final report each one gives before going off duty. At that time, by referring to the care plans and your own work plan, you should make certain that all aspects of nursing care and all additional duties have been completed. Record important observations on the patient's charts. Relay this information to the head nurse and to the oncoming team leaders.

Before your day is finished, you must evaluate the effectiveness of your own leadership and the nursing care given by your team. Determine how well the team worked together. Look back over the day's work for any areas that could have been improved. Finally, you must plan for tomorrow.

STUDY QUESTIONS

1. Select a problem. Using the five steps of problem-solving, try to arrive at a suitable solution.
2. Observe one person as she does her work. Determine specific activities that show good work organization. Select areas that show poor organization and indicate how they can be improved.
3. Plan the individual assignments for a typical team assigned to care for an average group of patients. How are the individual needs of the patients assigned? How is this information given to the team? How did you determine the sequence of duties? How is this indicated to each team member? How are the capabilities of each team member, including the team leader, utilized?
4. List as many factors as possible that will stimulate a spirit of cooperation within the team.
5. What personal qualities in the team leader aid cooperation?
6. How much responsibility can be assumed by a team member for planning her own work?
7. What administrative functions does the team leader use during this period of preparation?
8. Select a specific idea which someone you know believes. Try to persuade this person to change his beliefs concerning this idea. How will you know if you have succeeded?
9. What specific information should be included for a recently employed practical nurse and nurses' aide on your station during orientation as given by a team leader?
10. What are the characteristics of a good patient report? What information should be included?
11. What are the characteristics of a good assignment?
12. Observe several people as they give directions. Pick out methods used that you consider to be good. Pick out any mistakes and determine how they could have been avoided.
13. Make out a complete work plan when you are assigned to give patient care.
14. What helpful suggestions could you give to an individual who is having difficulty in organizing her work?
15. Give the various reasons why some people are unable to complete their assignments on time?
16. Prepare a time schedule for any shift, showing the time sequence of a team leader's activities.

6

HOW TO SUPERVISE YOUR TEAM

The aim of team nursing is the improvement of nursing care by means of more professional help and guidance for nonprofessional personnel. This help and guidance, or supervision if one wants to call it that, is very different from, and can never take the place of, that which the head nurse and supervisor must give. The basic principles and methods, however, remain the same.

SUPERVISION AND THE TEAM LEADER

Today nonprofessional personnel give much of the bedside care to the patient. Theirs is largely an on-the-job training in following set procedures for certain routine tasks. Thus, the more help, encouragement, and guidance they receive, the better able they will be to do good work. There is a direct relationship between the help they receive and the quality of the care they are able to give. In other words, the care given by nonprofessional workers will be only as good as the help, or supervision they receive.

Just as the nonprofessional person needs help to do her job, so also do the team leader, the nursing student, the head nurse, and others. In fact, in any position there comes a time when the person needs advice and guidance from someone more experienced than she. Supervision then can be described as *guided learning*.

In fact, Cecilia Perrodin,* in *Supervision of Nursing Service Personnel,* defines nursing supervision as "a service devised to improve patient care by the promoting, stimulating, and fostering of personnel growth and welfare."

Everyone should welcome this kind of supervision. First, however, nurses themselves must change their ideas of what supervision is and consequently their methods of giving it. The old-fashioned belief that a supervisor is one who commands and inspects has no place in the new concept of nursing supervision. The nursing profession is stressing the right of the patient to be considered an individual and to receive care that is based on his own particular needs. However, the nursing profession has not yet made much progress toward accepting the idea that each employee, especially the nonprofessional worker, has the same right to be considered an individual who is able to contribute to the effectiveness of the organization. Team nursing is a step in this direction.

Administration has been defined earlier as "the direction or management of a group of people"; supervision has been defined as "a tool through which administration becomes effective." Consequently, any person who works with and directs the activities of others must apply both the principles of administration and those of supervision. Since the team leader is concerned with directing the activities of her team, she is also responsible for supervising them in their work.

LEGAL ASPECTS OF TEAM LEADERSHIP

It is almost impossible to give specific information about the legal aspects inherent in the practice of team nursing. Although every state has a nursing practice law, each state sets its own standards and often does not define, except in general terms, what constitutes the practice of professional nursing or of practical nursing. Consequently, the interpretation and practice of nursing functions and responsibilities and the standards of care may vary from area to area within a state as well as throughout the nation.

Every nurse is, first of all, a citizen and, as a citizen, must be willing to assume the responsibilities imposed by law. Although nursing practice laws do benefit the nurse, they are mainly concerned with the protection of people. In nursing, as in few other professions, the practitioner is directly responsible for the safety and welfare of people; therefore, the nurse must be well informed

---

*Perrodin, Cecilia M. *Supervision of Nursing Service Personnel.* The Macmillan Company, New York, 1957, page 1.

about the ways of meeting her legal obligations in the practice of her profession within her own state and community.

According to Lesnik and Anderson, seven areas have been legally identified as professional nursing activities. In the area involving the execution of the physician's orders the nurse's activities may be considered to be dependent; however, in the other areas she is an independent practitioner. Today the registered nurse is finding that one of her major responsibilities is the direction and supervision of the allied health personnel who give patient care; therefore, she must recognize that she may be liable if her actions result in another person acting in a negligent manner. The professional nurse may be liable not only for the injurious acts of her agents, e.g., the practical nurse, done within the scope of authority but also for her failure to carry out her legal responsibility of directing and supervising the care of the patient, including that given by licensed practical nurses and other health workers.

Legal Responsibility for Planning the Nursing Care of the Patient. As has been stated several times previously and certainly implied by Lesnik and Anderson, the professional nurse must give care which goes beyond mere execution of the doctor's orders or adherence to hospital policy. In this area she has the duty to render that quality and quantity of care as given by the average nurse in the community at that time. This care must be planned and is based upon the nurse's application of principles found in the biologic, the physical and the social sciences.

This plan of care necessitates the assessment of the patient's nursing needs, the making of a nursing diagnosis, the determination of appropriate nursing measures, and the execution of the plan in order to achieve the aim of nursing care.

All of these are professional nursing activities and are essential in team leadership. The team leader together with her team members determines an appropriate plan of nursing care for each patient during the team conference. When put into written form, the care plan provides the team with a constant reminder and guide about what they hope to accomplish for the patient. It also provides the team leader with a basis for evaluating both the care of the patient and the work of each team member. Without the use of these tools, the nursing staff cannot truthfully say that they are using team nursing.

Legal Implications Related to the Assignment of Patient Care. Concern for the safety and well-being of the patient is of primary importance when assignments are made. Job titles such as nurses' aide, or even licensed practical nurse, do not indicate the degree of skill or understanding of the individual. Failure of the leader to recognize this may make her liable for injury caused by an act of one of her subordinates. The team leader must consider the needs of the patient, the capabilities of her team members, and the policies of the organization when making assignments to perform nursing techniques or to execute any therapeutic treatments which she may delegate to other personnel.

An important aspect in making assignments involves the manner in which they are given. Each person must understand exactly what she is to do, thus defining the scope of authority of the subordinates or agents and, consequently, limiting the liability of the professional nurse. Errors in giving treatments or doing any part of the patient's care may occur when directions do not indicate clearly who is to perform the care or what and how it is to be done. Every team member should receive a complete report about her patients and an explanation of her assignment before beginning her day's work.

Responsibility To Provide Supervision. Negligence may result from acts of omission as well as acts of commission. The law defines *direction* broadly as governing, ruling, or ordering and *supervision* as overseeing or inspecting. Gradually, nursing is accepting a broader definition of supervision, perhaps implied in the term *overseeing,* to include teaching and guidance of the worker to help him to do his best. This broader definition implies that a qualified person observes the worker and helps and teaches him whenever the need is observed. The responsibility related to assignment of patient care is not discharged until the care is completed in the way the team leader desires. To insure completion of all assignments she must supervise each team member during as well as after the giving of patient care.

Legal Responsibility Involving Observing and Reporting Responses of the Patient and Evaluating Nursing Care. Here the team leader has a professional and legal obligation to use all information obtained by her team. One of the major differences between the professional nurse and the allied nursing personnel is the ability and obligation of the professional nurse to interpret and evaluate facts and decide upon the appropriate action.

The team leader must demand and get all the information she can about each patient; therefore, she must help her team members to learn what to observe and must impress upon them the importance of reporting their observations and findings to her. She may wish to verify these observations before taking final action, but she is legally responsible for her use of all the information that is brought to her attention. Obtaining and using such information, whether to help in planning the care of a patient or in evaluating the care already given, is an important part of a team leader's supervisory responsibility.

No specific criteria can be set down by which negligence may be determined. In general, negligence may be shown if the nurse fails to exercise due care or demonstrates lack of reasonable skill in her performance compared to that expected of a nurse with similar education and experiences in that community at the time of the specific incident.

The team leader must keep informed about hospital policies, including job descriptions for herself and her team members. There is always an element of danger when someone says, "We always do it this way." All policies and job descriptions should be in writing and kept up-to-date so that there is never any question concerning what should and should not be done, thus helping to protect both the employing agency and the employee.

Each individual is held liable for her own acts, whether she is a registered nurse, a licensed practical nurse, a nursing student, or a nurses' aide. The professional nurse, however, has a moral obligation, although not a legal one, to help each worker to understand her legal obligations toward the patient.

Team members will learn by watching the team leader; therefore, the team leader must be careful that she always demonstrates high standards of nursing practice, ethically as well as legally. She should help her team members to understand their legal obligations involving making medical diagnoses, offering opinions about treatment, slander, and invasion of privacy, especially concerning confidential information. In these areas the team leader can teach both by her actions and by giving specific information.

SUPERVISION IS THE KEY TO TEAM LEADERSHIP

If we accept the fact that the team leader must direct and help the members of her team improve their skill to give good nursing care, then supervision becomes the key to effective team leadership, for, in democratic supervision, the supervisor must be a leader, "going before as a guide." It would seem then that the techniques used in leadership are a necessary part of supervision.

Supervision by the team leader starts when the report is given and the assignment explained, and continues until the team member is told of her progress and is helped to improve in her work. Supervision uses information and skills from many areas — teaching, communication, evaluation and guidance, and human relations. Since the team leader works closely with the members of her team, she should make use of these skills to insure good nursing care as she guides and directs her group in the care of their patients. In addition, she should be able to stimulate her team to improve patient care, not because they must, but because they want to.

SUPERVISION USES TEACHING

Supervision in itself is not teaching, yet it must make use of some of the teaching skills as a means of helping the worker. This can be done easily and effectively while the team leader works with her team.

What Is Learning? Learning does not always insure the acquisition of understanding and wisdom. Funk and Wagnalls define *learning* as "the process of getting knowledge," and *knowledge* as "the aggregation of facts and principles, acquired and retained," thus implying that a certain amount of active participation on the part of the learner is necessary. *Wisdom* and *understanding,* on the other hand, imply the ability to put knowledge into practice through the use of judgment and the power to make decisions.

Some Fallacies Concerning Teaching. Two fallacies concerning teaching need to be considered. The first involves the belief that when all the facts and information have been presented, learning has taken place and the teacher's work is finished. Frequently, when trying to determine the reason for an error, a teacher may exclaim, "But I *taught* her how to do it!" What this teacher really means is, "I *told* her how to do it." The mere giving of a certain amount of information in no way guarantees the learning of it; learning will not occur unless the learner wishes to acquire that knowledge. Certainly the ability to repeat the information, thus acquired, does not, in itself, indicate understanding, which is the ability to apply knowledge in a practical way.

Schools of nursing often emphasize the acquisition of knowledge but pay little attention to the degree of understanding that the nursing student acquires or needs. Most examinations in nursing are objective in form and stress recognition of facts, rather than the application of those facts to a particular patient. The so-called situation questions are difficult to make, especially those that will give a valid evaluation of a student's understanding of an actual nursing problem. Yet the acquisition of this understanding is extremely important if we are to have well-prepared nurses, capable of assuming leadership roles either in team nursing or in other fields of nursing.

A teacher can never assume that what she thinks she has taught and what the student has actually learned are the same. One day while supervising her students, a nursing instructor saw one student bathing a patient who was inadequately draped. The instructor discussed the reasons for draping, and the student indicated her knowledge of the various acceptable methods that could be used. Several days later the teacher came into a room while this same student was again bathing a patient who was incorrectly covered. The student's explanation was, "I didn't think you were coming around today!" The instructor thought she had taught the student to cover all her patients correctly. Actually, the student had learned only that she must cover the patient whenever the instructor was observing her.

Another common fallacy concerns the belief that teaching can be done only in a classroom. Nothing can be farther from the truth. Teaching and learning can occur at any time and in any place. Probably one of the most important methods of teaching is by example; people learn from watching and listening to others. Attitudes, ideas, beliefs, even ways of doing things, are passed on from one person to another in this way. The adage, "What you do speaks so loudly I can't hear what you say," is especially true in nursing. Those methods of nursing care that a person observes and practices on the hospital wards will be remembered much longer than the methods described, or even demonstrated, in the classroom. A graduate nurse will often say, "I could never be a teacher," yet the staff nurse is one of the most important teachers in nursing today because others will do as they see her do. Many a woman has learned to make a bed correctly while she was a patient in the hospital. Moreover, in team nursing, the members of the team will watch their leader and will follow her example as they care for their patients.

The Results of Learning. The end result of learning is a change in behavior and may involve mental, emotional, or physical activity. In other words, learning may change either a person's thoughts and ideas, his attitudes, or his ways of doing things. The manifestations of these changes will vary according to the individual's capacity or opportunity for self-expression and will not be noted until a situation arises in which that learning must be used. A person may respond in a certain way because of the teaching he received weeks, months, or even years previously. Learning took place at that time, but the evidence of his learning did not appear until he had occasion to apply his knowledge.

Four Steps To Use in Teaching. As team leader, you will need to apply your entire knowledge of medical therapy and nursing principles as you try to improve the care of your patients. You will need to increase your understanding of people and their reactions, not only of your patients but of your team members and of yourself as well. In addition, you will need to use various methods of teaching to help your group to acquire more knowledge and understanding of what good nursing care entails.

The four main steps to effective teaching are *prepare, present, practice,* and *follow-up.* Each step is important and leads naturally into the following one.

PREPARE. This includes the preparation of the learner as well as the preparation of yourself as teacher. First of all, you should decide what you want the person to learn. Go over the sequence of points in your own mind or jot them down in the form of a written outline. Make certain that all material is arranged in logical order. You must give some thought also to the prerequisite knowledge that is necessary if the person is to understand what you hope to teach. Decide how you want to present your information. Don't use the same method all the time. Have all the necessary equipment available before you begin. Of course, it goes without saying that you must know your subject.

After you have decided *what* and *how,* you must find out how much the learner knows about the subject already, or what background knowledge she has. For example, it would be difficult to teach someone how to measure output if she does not understand the meaning of cc. or oz. on measuring devices. Start with that which she knows, and proceed to the unknown. Always try to relate the information to what she already understands. Because a procedure is routine or the information is simple to you, do not assume that it will be routine or simple to someone else.

Try to put the person at ease, physically as well as emotionally. External distractions should be minimized as much as possible. At the same time, you should try to show the learner why she needs to know the material being presented and how it will help her in her work. In other words, try to arouse her interest in the subject. Learning occurs with greater rapidity when the learner is receptive, i.e., at ease and interested.

PRESENT. This second step is made up of two parts—telling and showing. Sometimes the discussion may precede the demonstration. Often, however, they are combined into a single operation, but both steps should be used to make your teaching more understandable.

Consider first how to present by telling. Here you must use all the techniques previously discussed in relation to communication—both verbal and nonverbal. Use simple terms that can be understood by the learner. There is no need to show off your complete knowledge of the subject. A good teacher knows how to sort out and use only that information needed by the learner. Giving too much explanation might cause confusion, thereby retarding the learning process.

Make your instruction personal to the learner, repeatedly telling her how she can make use of it. Use illustrations familiar to her, yet ones that are related to the new material being presented. For instance, if you are describing a new method for preventing bedsores, show her how one of her own patients could be helped by this method.

Another important part in the presentation is determining that the person understands what you are telling her, and that she is interpreting what you say correctly. If she does not seem to understand, be patient. Whenever it is necessary to repeat, try a different approach, using different words either to define the terms that were not understood or to restate the information. Technical abbreviations or medical terminology, such as hemiplegia or mediastinum, may not be completely understood by a young nursing student or a nonprofessional person, even though they may use them quite glibly. Unless you are trying to teach the meaning and correct usage of terms, try to avoid using very technical language.

Always put in positive terms those things that the person is expected to do; use the negative, i.e., things not to do, when you want to emphasize precautions necessary for the safety of the patient. In both cases, you should give a brief and simple explanation of the purpose of the procedures or the reasons for the treatment the patient is receiving. It is very important that the person, especially the nonprofessional person, should gain an adequate understanding of the total care that the patient needs.

A seriously injured accident victim, who had a tracheostomy to facilitate suctioning, was admitted to a surgical ward. The team leader asked a nurses' aide to help her in the care of this patient and then instructed her in giving her part of the care. Later the nurse was shocked to overhear this nurses' aide exclaim to another aide, "If I am ever hurt, I don't want to come to this hospital. The first thing they do is slit your throat!" Clearly this aide did not understand the importance of the tracheostomy in the treatment of this patient. Furthermore, she would probably discuss her feelings not only with hospital personnel but also with people outside the hospital, thereby creating a problem in public relations. Perhaps a few additional words by the team leader as the two worked together would have increased the aide's understanding and, consequently, her appreciation of the treatment necessary for this patient.

However, explanation alone is sometimes not enough. Verbal illustrations, while helpful, cannot take the place of visual aids; therefore, demonstration is also an important aspect of teaching, especially in team nursing. The power of your setting the example has already been mentioned and may be described as an informal demonstration of nursing care or behavior that others will observe and perhaps learn. Visual aids definitely help to develop a better understanding of information and foster retention of facts. They may be used to demonstrate ways of giving certain aspects of patient care, or to explain reasons for doing the care in a certain way. Examples of visual aids that you could use to make your teaching more interesting and understandable include pictures, models, sample equipment, or demonstrations of a procedure itself.

When giving a demonstration, go through it slowly, taking one step at a time. Additional explanation should be given throughout, even though you may have given some preliminary information already. Show the easiest way to do the procedure, stressing the precautions and reasons for doing each step. This explanation should not be lengthy nor be given in technical terms. Keep in mind that the simpler the explanation, the easier it will be for the learner to understand and remember it.

Place the learner so that she can see clearly each step of the demonstration and preferably from the same angle as when she does it herself. In other words, if you are teaching someone how to tie a square knot, the person should be watching from behind you rather than facing you, so that your movements and the appearance of the knot will not be reversed.

Allow time for comments and questions. When the procedure is difficult or long, repetition will probably be necessary. The fact that the learner does not ask questions does not always indicate understanding. Sometimes her lack of comprehension is so great that she is unable to ask questions, or she may think she understands when in reality she does not. Therefore, you should ask a few questions yourself to determine if you are getting your information across.

PRACTICE. Doing a procedure, or putting the information into practice, is a necessary step in the learning process. It also gives you the opportunity to check the correctness of the person's learning. At first, this practice must be done under your supervision, the closeness of which will be determined by the past experience of the individual and by the complexity of the procedure. Do not offer too much assistance in the actual performance. It is usually best to suggest the correct method rather than taking over and doing it yourself. For example, you may suggest:

    Don't you think it would be easier if . . . ?
    Remember there is something else that should be done first.
    Do you remember what I did next?
    Now stop and think a minute before you do that.

The average person needs several such practice periods in order to develop manual dexterity and to remember the proper sequence of steps necessary for a given procedure. Encourage the learner as she shows improvement and gains in self-confidence. The amount of help and direction may be decreased as the worker shows evidence of learning; however, a certain amount of supervision will always be necessary. You can never leave your team members to practice entirely on their own.

FOLLOW-UP. Additional checking at intervals is a necessary and important aspect of teaching. Observe the individual as she performs the entire procedure; look at the finished product; ask some questions to determine if she remembers the reasons for giving the care and the precautions necessary for the safety of the patient. Suggest ways in which she can improve but be very sure to compliment her on the part of her performance that she did well.

This discussion may make the teaching of good nursing care seem lengthy and a somewhat complicated process; however, this is not true. For example, suppose that, as you are passing out medications, you observe a nurses' aide trying to release the side rails on a patient's bed. They are new and somewhat different from the ones previously used, and she is unable to remove them. She is already in a situation that has prepared her for being taught; you need only to introduce your instruction by saying, "Let me help you." Your presentation of the method and its demonstration may consist of, "To lower this side rail, just remove these two pins. This unlocks the rail. Now you can fold it together like this. Then fasten it here so that the rail is out of the way. Just to be safe, always press down on the rail to make sure that it is locked securely." She watches while you lower the rail and lock it in place, then she goes around to the other side of the bed and releases the other rail. This is her practice period. You have taught; she has learned. The time involved was probably not over three minutes.

Perhaps you overhear one of your group saying, "I don't see why we have to get old Mr. Jones up in a chair every day. All we do is lift him from one place to another." Here is a good opportunity to do some teaching by answering the implied question, and thus increasing the understanding of the purpose for this aspect of the patient's treatment in relation to his needs. You can give the information immediately, or you can bring the incident up during the discussion at a team conference so that the entire group will benefit from the explanation.

Teaching, including the subsequent follow-up or observation, is fundamental to good supervision. Each member of your team must know what she is to do and how to do it. It is your responsibility to give her the opportunity to acquire this knowledge whenever she needs it. Teaching may also be necessary to help the person acquire acceptable attitudes, better appreciation of her place on the team, and a clearer understanding of her responsibility to the patient.

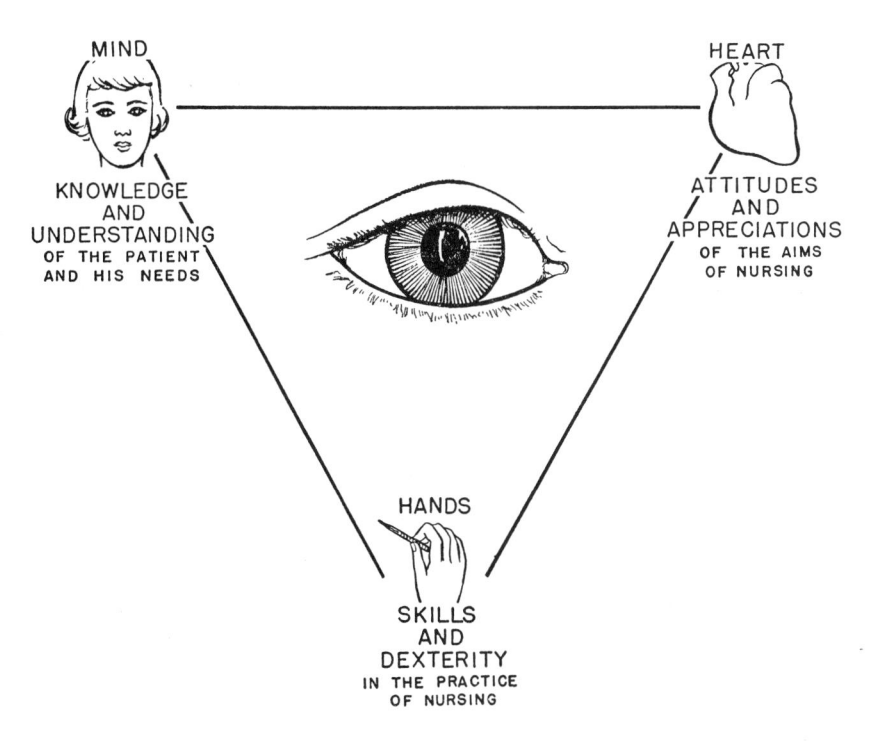

Figure 4. Areas to be supervised
The mind and the heart must guide the hands in the practice of nursing. Adapted from Perrodin, Cecilia: Supervision of Nursing Service Personnel. *The Macmillan Company, 1957.*

WHAT AREAS SHOULD BE SUPERVISED?

Cecilia Perrodin* suggests in her book, *Supervision of Nursing Service Personnel,* that three elements are necessary in good supervision. These are the *mind,* which gives an insight into supervision and its aims and functions, the *hand,* which puts into practice the art of supervision and, last but not least, the attitudes and appreciations, which are the *heart* of supervision.

These same elements also suggest the areas that need to be observed during supervision, because the *mind* and the *heart* guide the *hand* in the giving of good nursing care, and one cannot be separated from the others. All too often concern is shown only

---

*Perrodin, Cecilia M.: *Supervision of Nursing Service Personnel.* The Macmillan Company, New York, 1957, page 29.

about the correctness of detail and the manual dexterity demonstrated in the performance of care given by the individual, while little, if any, consideration seems to be given to the degree of empathy or understanding manifested by the worker for the patient. Each area is important, for each shows a different ability of the worker and, when combined, indicate her ability to understand and give total patient care. When separated, they provide only fragments of information; together they disclose the person as a complete individual. How then can you supervise so that all areas are included in your observation of each member of your team?

TECHNIQUES OF OBSERVATION

As a tool of administration, the process of supervision makes use of different, although interrelated, activities. Planning and organizing, making assignments, and teaching have already been discussed. Now comes the follow-up, which is done by observing your team in action. This observation involves more than just inspection and checking, although these are important. Observation, as used here, implies the acquisition of information through the use of all of your senses, including your intuition, sometimes called the sixth sense. You should observe continuously, while you look, do, talk, listen, write, and read. The process of evaluation should be carried on simultaneously with observation.

Learn To See What You Look At. Have you ever looked for a pencil, your bandage scissors, or a certain instrument and been unable to locate it, only to have it suddenly appear in front of you? You know that it was there all the time, and you had probably looked at it many times during your search, yet you could not see it. This can happen to you also as you observe your team members. However, through conscious effort, you can increase your ability to see. Here are some suggestions that may help you learn to see what you look at

HAVE SOME IDEA WHAT TO LOOK FOR BEFORE YOU BEGIN YOUR OBSERVATION. In order to do this, you will need to use all the knowledge you have gained in your entire classroom and clinical experience. Ask yourself continuously what and how, for example:
1. What symptoms should I look for in this patient?
2. What safety measures should be used for this patient? Are they being used?
3. How should the patient's environment appear when his care has been completed?

4. What is each member of my team doing at this moment?
5. Is the nurses' aide turning the patient often enough? What method is she using?

Be careful to look at every aspect of the patient's care and environment; this will include the care he is receiving and has already received. However, do not concentrate on single details only and thus neglect to obtain an over-all picture of the patient's care and his response to it. Keep in mind other information that can be obtained through what you see, for example, the sympathy shown toward the patient, or the method of adapting the principles of a procedure to fit a particular need of a patient, thereby indicating an understanding and appreciation of the patient's problems by the worker. Keep checking back on the questions you want answered, although you do not want to limit yourself to that information only, as you watch your team in action.

CONSIDER EACH PERSON AS AN INDIVIDUAL. If you are to determine what to observe in the care of a patient, you will need to give some thought to his individual needs. When you observe one of your team members at work, you will need to compare the care she is giving with that which she is capable of giving. In like manner, you will need to consider her attitudes, her emotions, and her differences. It is impossible to pour everyone into the same mold by expecting them to think alike, to act alike, or to give nursing care in exactly the same way. Your understanding of the individual should give you more self-confidence in your personal relations with her. Furthermore, a greater spirit of cooperation follows the consideration of the personal desires, needs, and abilities of the individual.

TRY TO BE OBJECTIVE ABOUT WHAT YOU SEE. If ten people observe a certain incident and then try to describe it, there will probably be ten different versions. Everyone will have his own interpretation of the incident and is sure in his own mind that he saw it happen that way. There are several reasons why it is sometimes difficult to get a factual account of any incident.

First of all, a person fails to be objective in his observations because his attitudes and motives may cause him unconsciously to overlook or to exaggerate certain things. It is not uncommon for a person to see only what he wants to see. It may be extremely difficult for an individual to be entirely objective when observing someone whom he either likes or dislikes intensely. Since what the individual believes he sees is often controlled by his preconceived ideas, beliefs, or emotions about the situation in general, he may generalize and then look for examples to prove that he is correct. For example, if a person believes that all teen-agers are juvenile delinquents, he will see only those incidents that tend to support his belief. He will either fail to look for or to recognize anything contrary to his belief.

Another reason for this lack in objectivity lies in the fact that a person's mind tends to supply that part of the action which he did not see, thus making those facts which he did observe meaningful to him. For instance, as a nurse passes the door of a patient's room, she hears a noise and turns in time to see the patient pulling himself up into a chair from a kneeling position on the floor. Unless she is aware of the legal implications, she will probably say that the patient fell out of bed. Yet, when she is asked, she will be unable to say truthfully that she saw the actual fall. Her belief that he fell stems from the fact that she filled in an action that might have caused the noise she heard, and which would have accounted for the position of the patient when she first saw him.

When a person realizes the importance of being objective in his observations, he will also realize that he must obtain all the facts before he is justified in drawing any conclusion. Assuming that something has happened or that something is true without first obtaining substantiating evidence invalidates any conclusion based on those assumptions. Conclusions should be made only after all the facts have been collected.

As team leader, try to be accurate and objective in your observations of both your patients and the members of your team. Try to obtain all the facts. For example, you should be careful in believing that a team member did not do a certain part of her assignment simply because she has been known to omit it in the past. On the other hand, you are not justified in thinking that someone has completed her work simply because she has always done so in the past. You must have sufficient evidence before drawing any conclusions. The fact that one of your team members neglected on one day to tell you about the symptoms of one of the patients does not justify your saying that she usually fails to observe symptoms accurately, that she usually forgets to report them, or, as is so often the remark if this person is a nursing student, that she does not assume responsibility.

The knowledge that your attitudes and emotions are likely to color what you see should make you especially careful in making your observations. When you feel irritable and tired, you are likely to pick up those incidents that provoke you; when you feel happy, you will tend to overlook these same incidents.

LOOK FOR RELATIONSHIPS OR ASSOCIATIONS BETWEEN WHAT YOU SEE AND WHAT THE OVER-ALL SITUATION APPEARS TO BE. Any incident is made up of a number of separate actions, each of which could have a number of different meanings when separated from the total incident. Therefore, it is necessary to observe not only individual steps of nursing care but also to consider each step in relation to total care needed by the patient. Do not look for errors only, but consider the entire performance of the worker. Seeing how all aspects of care fit together will indicate, to some extent, the understanding that the worker has concerning the needs of her patient. You should determine if each part of the care is correctly given, but you should also observe whether the proper sequence of steps or procedures is used.

BE INTERESTED IN WHAT YOU SEE. Interest helps you to be more complete and accurate in your observation of details. This can be demonstrated in your ability to recognize a person and remember his name. If, at the time of your introduction to this person, you were extremely interested in him and anxious to meet him, you will later be able to describe him quite accurately and will be able to recognize him the next time that you see him. If, however, you were busy thinking of other things and gave only superficial attention at the time of the introduction, you will find it extremely difficult to remember specific details about the individual, because you did not really see those details in the first place.

Interest in your patients and in the nursing care given by your team will increase your ability to see what your team members are doing, because you will tend to give greater attention to the details of their work. Concentration while consciously looking for details will also help you to see better. You can never allow yourself to become so engrossed in your own work and in your own problems that you look at, but are unable to see, the work and problems of others.

Learn To Listen. Perhaps the biggest obstacles to effective team leadership lie in talking too much and forgetting to listen. Learn to listen to what others are saying. Group feeling is stimulated when each member feels free to offer suggestions, knowing that you will give them thoughtful consideration. Remember that your position as team leader does not give you the right to do all the planning, make all the suggestions, or issue only commands. Resentment is usually the end result of such autocratic leadership, and instead of welcoming your supervision, the worker will tend to avoid it and you, whenever possible.

Some of the aspects of listening were discussed in the section on communication. As a reminder, however, remember that you need to listen for the "overtones" in a person's conversation. It is not always what is said that counts. The tone or inflection of voice along with the facial expressions are important in giving meaning to the spoken words. Look at the person while she is speaking. Give her time to express herself and indicate your interest in what she is saying. Listen as she talks with the other members of the team or with her patients. Ask yourself if the information she is giving is correct, if she is displaying the proper understanding of the patient and of the care he needs, and if she shows an appreciation of his problems.

Every team leader must spend time with her patients—looking and listening. All too often nurse-patient communication is nurse-directed. Commonly it consists of comments about the weather—past, present, and future—or the casually asked question, "How are you this morning?" Directions and information are given in the same offhand manner, and the patient feels that the nurse is not interested in him personally. Most conversations can be patient-directed, although there are times when the nurse may need to steer the conversation toward various other channels. The patient should always be allowed to choose the topic of conversation; the nurse merely helps him to express or identify his feelings. She indicates her interest without showing disapproval and without making decisions for him. She gives information when necessary or may offer suggestions, when these seem needed, to help the patient solve his problem. But whatever the trend of the conversation, the nurse cannot ignore what the patient wants to talk about.

Learn To Use Your Other Senses. While your sense of taste may play a minor part in your observations, you should learn to use your senses of smell and touch to add to your information about the care your patients need or are receiving. Are there unpleasant odors? What can be done about getting rid of them? Is this patient particularly sensitive to odors? Do certain odors convey pleasant or unpleasant ideas to the patient? For example, the odor of certain flowers reminded one patient of the death and funeral of his wife and caused him to become very depressed. Does the foundation of the bed look smooth, but more than that, does it feel smooth? Is the temperature of the room or of the bath water too warm or too cool for the patient? With practice you will find many other areas for using your senses of touch and smell.

Cultivate Your Intuition. This sixth sense comes with experience. You get a certain feeling, nothing definite, nothing that is the result of a logical thought process. It is the result of the knowledge and understanding you have accumulated from your various experiences in similar situations. While you cannot rely upon your intuition alone, you cannot ignore its presence. Perhaps the thought occurs that you should check on a certain patient. Do so; it could be important. Something tells you that not all the pertinent information has been given about a certain situation; keep searching until you are satisfied.

Observe Continuously. Although you should observe your team constantly, you do not want to watch any individual too closely.

Constant observation is not necessarily close observation. The first gives the worker a sense of confidence and security; the other indicates your lack of confidence and trust in her ability to do her work. The purpose of observation is to give you a source of information that you can use to guide, help, and encourage your team in their work. Observation is also necessary to determine the effectiveness of the nursing care given by your team.

Of course, good observation can be done only when you know what to look for and how to see it. This means, as discussed previously, an adequate knowledge of the needs both of your patients and of your team, then an evaluation of what you see in order to determine how well the needs of both are being met. This knowledge can come only through personal contact with your patients and with your team, during which you consciously make use of all the techniques of observation.

OBSERVE AS YOU CARE FOR YOUR PATIENTS. One of the best times to observe your patient is during the time you are giving some of his care. Good rapport can be established at this time because he feels that you are doing something for him and, therefore, are interested in his welfare. Yet, how often have you seen a nurse enter a patient's room, carrying a trayful of medications, without seeming to give a thought to the patient himself? As she approaches the patient, she is busy checking the patient's name on the medicine card and the number of medicines she is to give him. When she reaches his bedside, she speaks his name or uses other means of identification, casually glancing at the patient as she does so. Perhaps she gives a word or two of instruction. Then, as she hands him the medicine and waits for him to take it, she looks again at her tray of medicines. She may glance once more at the patient, but chances are that she is thinking about the next patient rather than the one beside her. In such a situation, how much did the nurse see, hear, or feel about the patient and his environment?

As you do your work, learn to see your patient. Give your conscious attention to his expression, his color, his position in bed, his topics of conversation, and his environment. Compare what you expect to find with what you actually observe. In what aspects do differences appear? Are these differences significant to the patient's condition and to his general welfare?

OBSERVE AS YOU WORK WITH YOUR TEAM. It is generally unwise to stand by doing nothing except watching the person at work. This method of observation is the one that has caused the general belief that supervision is inspection. An opportune time to observe your team members is during the time you can work with one or more of them in caring for a particular patient. At this time, you can observe manual skills and ability to adapt steps of care to fit the patient's needs, as well as skill in communicating with the patient and his family. You should note whether the person attends to all the details of nursing care or omits some that she may feel are not important. Her attitude toward the patient may be manifested in her approach and manner toward him or in the way in which she gives the care itself.

OBSERVE DURING YOUR ROUNDS TO VISIT PATIENTS. During your morning rounds, you can gather some important information as you go from bedside to bedside; however, you will probably find it difficult to gain adequate information about personal problems because of lack of time. When you visit your patients at other times during the day, try to spend more time listening to them. One of the topics of conversation may be concerned with how the patient feels about the care he is receiving or about those who care for him.

The patient's evaluation of his care is important for two reasons. First, you are concerned with finding out how well your team is meeting the needs of each patient, and secondly, you may find areas in which the patient complains of a lack of care or is dissatisfied with his care. Public relations is one of your responsibilities, especially those public relations that begin with the care of the patient. As Monroe M. Title* comments in his article, *Public Relations Begin with the Patient:* "One dissatisfied, misinformed patient with an average number of friends can do much to injure the reputation and the good will of a hospital."

Much of the criticism of nurses and nursing care today arises because the patients and their friends and relatives do not understand the reasons for the care given or not given. For instance, people often think that getting up on the day of, or the day after, surgery is cruel. Usually they believe that the patient is permitted to get up early, allowed to go to the bathroom, and encouraged to give certain parts of his own care so that the hospital personnel will not have to do so much work. When the patient has this attitude, the aim of early ambulation may have been achieved, but the good will and respect of the patient have been lost. Actually, this criticism indicates the need for better communication and teaching in order to give the patient a better understanding, thereby gaining his active cooperation with the activities used to aid in his recovery.

OBSERVE AS YOU DO YOUR OWN WORK. Learn to weave your observation among and around your own duties. As you circulate or as you work, you have a chance unobtrusively to observe your team at work. Avoid giving the impression that you are snooping.

---

*Title, Monroe M.: *Public Relations Begin with the Patient.* Hospital Management, September, 1960, page 36.

However, you should be able to see how they are progressing with their individual assignments, what they are discussing with their patients and co-workers, their correctness in following established procedures and, perhaps, how they display their understanding of the patient.

OBSERVE DURING THE REPORT PERIOD. The report that each member of your team gives you at the completion of her assignment is a good source of information, not only about the patient and what was done for him but also about the attitudes and understanding of the person who gave that care. For example, when you get a report, you find out if all the work has been finished; at the same time, you can determine the worker's ability to follow directions and her interest in details. If the person is allowed to chart, still another source of information is available, for again you may find indications of the kind of work she does, whether it is hurried, slipshod, meticulous, neat, and so on. The spelling and content of her charting will also give you some idea about her interest in accuracy and the importance she attaches to this responsibility.

OBSERVE AFTER ALL CARE HAS BEEN GIVEN. You can continue to gain information about the work of your team if you visit the patients after their care has been completed. Suppose you enter the room of a patient who is suffering from heart decompensation and is on strict bed rest. You see that the window shade is arranged so that the morning sun shines in the patient's face. The patient himself is sitting up on the back rest, but the pillows are arranged so that his head is pushed forward onto his chest and his shoulders are hunched forward. His arms are lying outside the bed covers, which are pulled tightly across his chest, making it even more difficult for him to breathe. In addition, the sheet and spread hang unevenly down one side. The bedside table is pushed away from the bed. The water glass is half full of water that feels warm and looks stale. The signal cord is tucked under the pillow in such a way that the patient would have to exert himself to find it.

Contrast that picture with one you observe as you enter another room. This patient, a woman with far advanced cancer, is also sitting up in bed. Body alignment is good with the head, neck, and shoulders well-supported by pillows that are arranged correctly. The patient's hair is combed and tied with a bright ribbon. There is even a hint of lipstick and rouge. The bed covers are neat and arranged to give ample movement of the feet. The shades are fixed to give plenty of light and yet shut out any glare. On the over-the-bed table are fresh water, an open magazine, and a box of Kleenex. A paper bag for soiled tissues is pinned within easy reach of the patient. The signal cord is fastened so that the patient can reach it without turning. The tube from the retention catheter has plenty of slack yet is so arranged that the fluid will drain easily into a container.

It is obvious from these observations that you can get a great amount of information about the kind of care given to these two patients. You should not, however, render judgment on what you see only. Especially in the first case you should discuss with the worker what you observed and try to determine if there are valid reasons for the apparent poor care. You should also ask yourself some critical questions about your methods of making assignments and the amount of help given to the person who was assigned to care for this patient. Perhaps her assignment was too large for her ability to complete it, or she was interrupted too many times, or she was too inexperienced to care for this very ill patient.

Whenever you are observing, remember to consider what you can learn about the knowledge, understanding, and attitudes of those who are giving the nursing care.

HOW TO USE THE INFORMATION OBTAINED THROUGH OBSERVATION

In the supervision of your team, evaluation, like observation, must be a continuous process. All information obtained from your observation must be used to evaluate yourself and your team and to help each person to improve.

Evaluate Your Own Leadership and Supervision. Every leader must be able to criticize herself objectively and honestly, for until she is able to use self-criticism, she has no right to criticize others. She must be able and willing to improve herself, rather than offering excuses for her apparent weaknesses. Here are some examples of questions that may help in this self-evaluation:

1. Does your group accept your leadership?
2. Do you lead or do you "boss"?
3. Does your team welcome your help or do they seem to consider it interference?
4. How well are you helping your team to understand the meaning of good nursing care? Do areas appear where teaching is needed?
5. Do your team members follow your directions? How clear and specific are your directions? Do you include all the necessary information?
6. Are your assignments well-planned? Are you using the individual abilities of each person to the fullest extent?
7. Are you meeting the needs of the individual worker for recognition and security? Are you more concerned with the work or with the worker?

Evaluate the Understanding, Attitudes, and Performance of Your Team Members. If supervision is to be effective, you must use all the techniques of supervision, including evaluation of the work of each member of your team. If manual dexterity and correctness in doing procedures are the only aspects considered, you will be unable to help the worker to develop as an individual. Nursing care is more than the performance of procedures. Nursing care depends upon the relationship of nurse to patient; therefore, everyone must try to improve in the area of human relations in order to increase skill in getting along with people. Here are some examples of questions that will help in the evaluation of your team members:
1. Are they able to plan their work and complete their assignments?
2. Do they understand what is expected of them?
3. In what areas do they need to learn more?
4. How well do they follow procedures?
5. Do they tend to waste time and energy in any way? If so, why?
6. How does each person get along with the other members of her team? Does she prefer to work alone or with someone else?
7. What attitudes do they express about their patients?
8. Are the patients receiving good care? Are they satisfied with their care?

Evaluate the Team as a Whole. The team is made up of individuals; however, when there is a strong spirit of teamwork, the individuals cease to function independently and work together as one. Here are some examples of questions to help you to determine the effectiveness of the team as a unit:
1. Do the members of the group work together harmoniously?
2. Is the nursing care coordinated to meet the needs of the patient?
3. Is the group satisfied when their work is completed?
4. Does the team share in the planning of patient care? Does each one participate in group activities?
5. Do they express group consciousness through the use of the words, *we* and *our*?
6. Does the team look to you for leadership?

Help the Individual To Improve. If you are unable to help the person at the time of your observation, make a record of what you observed so that you can use it later in a conference with her. A written record concerning some observation about the person herself or about her work is called an *anecdotal note*. In some situations you, as a graduate nurse or as a team leader, may be asked to keep anecdotal notes on your team members to help the head nurse or supervisor evaluate the progress of the individual. It is not within the realm of this book to discuss the advisability of including this responsibility as part of the supervision of your team. However, since you may need to make these notes, a brief discussion of the elements necessary in a good anecdotal note will be included at this point.

ANECDOTAL NOTES MUST CONTAIN ONLY FACTUAL INFORMATION. Since an anecdotal note is a written record of an observation, all that has been said about making objective and accurate observations is true of the written record also. You must try to eliminate your feelings, interpretations, and evaluations as much as possible. One of the best ways to become objective in the recording of your observations is to answer the questions, "Who did it? What was done? To whom? And when?" In other words, include only what you saw or heard, so that when you talk with the individual later, you can give specific examples of her behavior or work.

A note which states, "Miss M. gave good nursing care this morning," is inadequate. This is an interpretation by the writer and the head nurse or supervisor who tries to summarize a number of such anecdotal notes will be unable to make her own evaluation of the performance of Miss M. Such a note may not be questioned since it indicates a good performance. But suppose the note reads, "Miss M. does not seem to understand children." Immediately, Miss M. will ask, "What makes you say that?" If the specific incident that caused this remark has not been included in the anecdotal note, the person doing the counseling will be unable to help Miss M. realize why she gives this impression. Instead of helping the person, such a note will only arouse her resentment.

OTHER INFORMATION IS NECESSARY TO COMPLETE THE NOTE. The date of the observation, and sometimes the specific time of the day, should be given in order to help the individual to recall the incident. The name of the person who was observed and the one who did the observing must also be included. Occasionally, to help the person doing the final summary or interpretation, the background of the incident can be given. For example, the fact that a large assignment was completed is not too significant in itself, but it does become important if all details of care were attended to even though the assignment included a number of very ill patients. Also the completion of such an assignment would be significant if the individual was usually unable to finish her work.

A SUFFICIENT NUMBER OF ANECDOTAL NOTES MUST BE AVAILABLE TO DETERMINE THE CHARACTERISTIC BEHAVIOR OF AN INDIVIDUAL. It is impossible to generalize on the basis of a single observation. The aim of anecdotal notes is to give an accurate composite picture of the individual, her skills, attitudes, and degree of understanding. In order to attain this, no incident is too small or too insignificant to be omitted from the record.

The fact that the worker went ahead and took afternoon temperatures without being reminded becomes important when other notes indicate that she took the initiative in emptying the linen hampers, straightening the service room, and so on. The fact that a person was very abrupt in answering the requests of a patient, or looked and spoke crossly, indicates her attitude or her emotions on one particular day only. Probably one of the main complaints made by personnel, especially by nursing students, about evaluation reports is the one, "How does she know how I usually do my work? She saw me only once." For this reason, an adequate number of good anecdotal notes is necessary. Characteristic behavior cannot be determined after seeing the individual do something one time only. A number of observations indicating similar behavior are necessary before the typical behavior of an individual can be determined.

ANECDOTAL NOTES MUST INCLUDE OBSERVATIONS OF BOTH THE STRONG AND WEAK ATTRIBUTES OF THE PERSON. All too often the only notations recorded are those that indicate what the worker did wrong. To be fair, an evaluation must show the strong points of the person as well as her weak areas. This means that the recorded observations must include this information. When the person is constantly criticized for her errors, and is given no indication that her work is satisfactory in any respect, she soon loses all interest in trying to improve. Giving recognition for good work is just as necessary, when helping a person to improve, as calling her attention to those areas in which she could do better.

As a team leader, you will not be asked to do counseling according to its usual definition. However, since one of your responsibilities in supervising your team is guiding and helping them, you will probably need to use some of the techniques of counseling as you work with them.

Every person has the right to know how she is doing. When she is kept informed of her progress, she is better able to realize what she should do to improve. Sometimes the information you obtain during your observation will need to be used immediately; sometimes the matter can be taken care of later. Whatever the time, you should take the person aside so that you can talk privately, especially if a reprimand or correction is necessary. Never under any circumstance "bawl out" an individual in front of her coworkers or a patient. The average person is interested in learning how she can do her work better. She is always pleased to learn that her good points are recognized or that her work is satisfactory and appreciated. There is perhaps justification for the complaint,

"The only time I find out how I am doing is after I do something wrong." A very important method of gaining the cooperation of your group is getting them to realize that you will give honest praise, as well as correction, when they deserve it.

At first, you may find it difficult to talk to anyone of your group about her work. You will find that a better feeling will exist if you praise first then offer correction afterward. It may also be easier to begin if you have some general opening sentences to use, for instance you could begin with:

"I would like to say how well you . . ."
"Some things which you do well are . . ."
"I have heard some very nice comments about your work."
"I liked the way you . . ."
"I want to let you know how much I appreciate . . ."
"Your . . . was very good (or was very well-done)."

Transitional phrases that you can use to approach your corrections and suggestions for improvement could be:

"However, I feel that . . ."
"However, I wonder about the report that . . ."
"Of course I realize that you started late (or some other extenuating circumstance) . . ."
"Now let's talk about . . ."
"There are some things that could be improved."

Throughout the discussion encourage the person to express her feelings or to offer her suggestions. You may want to say:

"What do you think about . . . ?"
"Do you think there is a better way of doing it?"
"Was there a reason for your doing it this way?"
"What would you suggest?"
"Am I correct in my facts?"

At the end of the conversation encourage the individual to put the recommended changes into practice immediately. To encourage such action you may say:

"I am sure you will find it better (or easier) if you . . ."
"Suppose you try it this way next time."
"I am sure that you will do better next time."
"If it happens again and you still have trouble, I'll be glad to help you."

SUPERVISION AND HUMAN RELATIONS

Developing Good Human Relations. Interpersonal or human relations are the result of the give and take between people; they are influenced by the interchange of thoughts and ideas — in other words, by communication. When communication is satisfactory, good human relations are more likely to develop. This does not mean total agreement. It does mean, however, that each person is sincere in trying to find the best way to reach a common goal and is, therefore, willing to work with others in attaining that goal.

If you want others to communicate with you, you must communicate with them. If you want cooperation, you must be cooperative. If you want respect, you must give respect. If you want to develop good human relations, you must set an example. Your recognition of the individual and her needs aids in winning her respect and loyalty. Fairness and impartiality are important in the development of good relations with other people. Keep an open mind; try to understand the other person's point of view. You should strive to win the respect of your group, not because your title of leader demands it but because your team realizes that you will help them to do the kind of work they can be proud of. They want to respect you not so much for the knowledge you possess but for the way in which you use it.

Each individual wants to feel that she is recognized as a person, not just a worker. You must try to meet the personal needs of each member of your team — her need for personal recognition, for security, for understanding, for the opportunity to use and develop her abilities, and for information about her relationship and contribution to the team and to the hospital. Try to give each one what industry is calling a "psychological pay check," i.e., the fulfillment of these needs. Sister Mary Margarella* gives fifteen words that influence the development of human relations:

    The five most important words are, "I am proud of you."
    The next four are, "What is your opinion?"
    The next three are, "If you please."
    The next two are, "Thank you."
    The smallest word in all the world is the pronoun, I.

Getting Along with Various Kinds of People. If your leadership is to be effective, you must be able to follow as well as to lead, to have confidence in others as well as in yourself, to be more interested in giving than in receiving, to help others and to let them help you. You must be able to work with all kinds of people.

The *average worker* is often overlooked. She does her assignment adequately, does not cause trouble, and is usually dependable; consequently, the team leader may fail to recognize this person's need for additional help.

You are responsible for helping each of your team members,

---

*Margarella, Sister Mary: *Communication: The Catalyst.* Hospital Progress, May, 1960, page 106.

including the one who is average. You must be able to stimulate her and assist her in developing her capabilities more fully. By so doing you will often find that an average worker can develop into a better than average, or even into a superior, worker.

The *superior worker* is sometimes neglected also because she seems capable of going ahead and of doing her work with less direction than the others. However, you cannot always assume that because a person is above average in some things, she will be above average in everything. There are always some areas where improvement can be encouraged. On the other hand, it is true that you can expect more of this person, and you should give her credit for her ability. This credit should not, however, take the form of an additional work load, but should be something that stimulates the individual to learn more, to become more skilled, or to assume more responsibility. This type of person is often bored with routine tasks; therefore, you need to plan her assignment carefully to provide the variety that will stimulate her to greater progress.

The *fast worker* is sometimes a superior worker who is able to plan more efficiently; however, this is not always true. Working too rapidly is more often the cause of errors than working too slowly; therefore, you will need to evaluate the quality of nursing care this person gives. If she omits details of care for the sake of saving time, you will need to help her to realize this weakness and show her how she can overcome it. On the other hand, if the quality of her work is good, you must show your recognition of her abilities, not by assigning more work, but rather by including in her assignment certain tasks that require more time and attention so that she becomes even more efficient.

The *slow worker* certainly needs your help. First of all, you will need to investigate to determine the reason for her slowness. Perhaps she is unable to plan her work to make the best use of her time. If this is the case, you will need to help her to learn to organize more efficiently. Sometimes the person who works slowly does so because she is of below average intelligence, which hinders thinking and planning ahead. Such an individual usually does well when assigned to routine tasks in which she can follow a procedure already developed. Perhaps there is a health problem that needs medical attention. On the other hand, she may be a person who tries to make all her work perfect, or she may be merely inexperienced and, therefore, unsure of herself.

The *perfectionist* is often an unhappy person in her job because of her frustration when unable to perform her work at the quality level she desires. She may either become disillusioned and quit, or else lose her ideals and assume a "don't care" or "so what" attitude. Neither response is desirable. Try to develop a satisfactory compromise between what she feels is the way care should be given and the way it can be given in a particular situation. This does not mean that she loses her ideals but rather that she sets her goals where she can reach them at the present time. Help her to understand what aspects of care are most important for each of her patients, then encourage her to do her best on those aspects, rather than trying to do everything for every patient.

The *inexperienced worker* needs close supervision until she gains more skill and knowledge. This help is necessary not only to insure safe nursing care but also to give her a feeling of security. You will need to plan her assignments to include both the aspects of care with which she is familiar and also new experiences, so that she will continue to learn. The speed with which you can add these new experiences will depend upon her ability to learn and gain understanding.

You may have on your team a very *aggressive person* who may try to get everything she wants and, if thwarted, may exhibit some other form of problem behavior, such as antagonism or argument. Some authorities believe that aggressive behavior is caused by frustration. Seek to understand the person. If possible, determine the reason for this behavior. On the other hand, you cannot afford to allow her to disrupt team spirit. Sometimes additional attention and honest praise, without giving in to her demands, will alleviate any feelings of insecurity or hostility she may have. Sometimes it is possible to discuss the situation frankly and arrive at an acceptable conclusion. Never argue with her; stick to the facts. Firm guidance is necessary if you are to maintain control. Above all else maintain your own self-control at all times.

The *overconfident person* also needs close supervision. Overconfidence is not the same as self-confidence. The individual who is capable of doing better than average work may be self-confident because she recognizes her capabilities and limitations and will not exceed them. On the other hand, the overconfident person is often unable to recognize her lack of knowledge and understanding and will, therefore, "rush in where angels fear to tread." You will need to give additional explanation to this person concerning what she is to do and what she must not do. You should also help her to increase her understanding of the patient, including how his care is to be given and why.

PROBLEMS THAT YOU CANNOT SOLVE

The head nurse has an important responsibility in team nursing. It is to her that you should turn for help and advice when situations develop that are beyond your ability to handle. Consult with her if you have difficulty arranging assignments, planning care for a particular patient, or encouraging teamwork and cooperation within your group. Personnel problems and rumors should always be reported to her so that she can deal with them properly.

QUESTIONS ASKED ABOUT SUPERVISION

How much supervision should be expected of the team leader? In order to increase her abilities in the field of administration, the team leader should be helped and encouraged to do as much supervision as she is capable of doing. We mean here, of course, that supervision which is the assistance and guidance of her team, necessary for good nursing care. Because of her close relationship with her team, the team leader has a better opportunity to give this kind of supervision than any other person who shares in this responsibility.

How can I overcome my reluctance to correct the members of my team? Perhaps part of your reluctance stems from your idea of how supervision is given. If you think of it as a means of helping your team while they are working, you may have less difficulty in showing them how to do better—whether it is because they are doing something incorrectly or because they should become more skillful in their work.

If you are a nursing student or a recent graduate and, therefore, feel reluctant because of your youth or lack of experience, I am

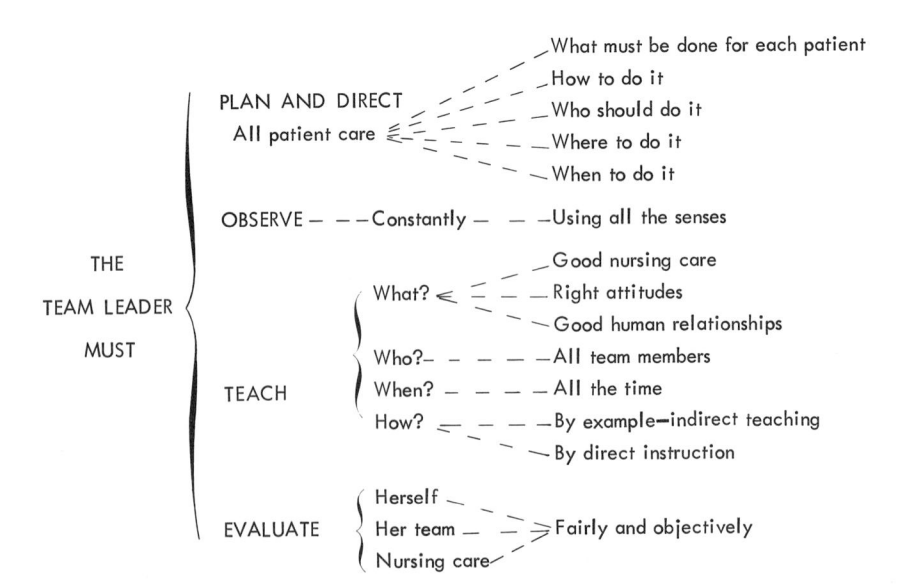

THE TEAM LEADER MUST
- PLAN AND DIRECT All patient care
  - What must be done for each patient
  - How to do it
  - Who should do it
  - Where to do it
  - When to do it
- OBSERVE — — Constantly — — —Using all the senses
- TEACH
  - What? — Good nursing care
    - Right attitudes
    - Good human relationships
  - Who? — — — —All team members
  - When? — — — — All the time
  - How? — — —By example—indirect teaching
    - By direct instruction
- EVALUATE
  - Herself
  - Her team — — Fairly and objectively
  - Nursing care

Figure 5. *Activities of the team leader.*

sure that this situation will correct itself in time. Meanwhile, whenever you try to help your team members improve, indicate to them that you are using information or techniques that your clinical instructors, supervisors, or head nurses have found helpful, thereby transferring some of their authority and experience to yourself. If a situation develops that you cannot handle, you should discuss the matter with your head nurse.

Should team nursing be practiced during all three shifts or only during the day shift? Team nursing can be used throughout the entire 24 hours, with each team having a conference and planning or revising nursing care plans. If you do not yet have team nursing on all shifts, you should make sure that the nursing care plans are used around the clock.

How can I follow these principles when the older graduates criticize and laugh at me? If the reader is one of those who has laughed at the enthusiasm and ideals of the nursing student or recent graduate and perhaps remarked, "It's all right to teach them that way, but wait until they get out on the station, they'll find out that things just don't work that way," then I hope you now realize how these nursing students classify you.

It is unfortunate that a nurse who wants to be considered a professional person is often opposed to trying new methods of giving nursing care, offering as her excuse, "It won't work." Instead, the professional nurse should be anxious to help, rather than undermine, any program that could improve nursing and maintain the ideals for which it stands.

On the other hand, I am sure that every instructor in nursing hopes that she can instill in her students such a keen desire to give good nursing care that they will have the stamina and strength to give nursing care in the way they believe it should be given, in spite of criticism or ridicule.

STUDY QUESTIONS

1. Compare the techniques of leadership with the activities carried on during supervision.
2. Why might the team leader be able to give better supervision, meaning help and guidance, than the head nurse or supervisor?
3. Discuss the statement that supervision might be defined as "guided learning."
4. Observe your own work as team leader, or the work of another leader. Select two instances of teaching. Determine how each of the four steps of teaching was carried out.
5. Check your ability to observe and remember details. Give yourself two minutes in a patient's room. At the end of the allotted time, list every specific observation about the patient and his environment you can remember. Answer as many as possible of the following questions, then return to the room and check the completeness and correctness of your observations.

a. What was the patient doing when you entered the room?
b. What was the patient's position?
c. What did the patient's mood appear to be?
d. In what position were the window curtains or shades?
e. Where was the patient's water glass? How much water was in it?
f. How tight were the bed covers over the patient's feet?
g. Did the light come from over the patient's left or right shoulder?
h. Where was the signal cord?
i. Answer the following if they apply: How many liters of oxygen was the patient receiving? How much fluid remained in the bottle of intravenous fluid? Were the drainage tubes arranged correctly?

6. Stage a highly dramatic incident in front of a group. Have each observer tell exactly what she saw. Check the results. Were there any differences in the various reports? Why did these occur?

7. Discuss methods by which a team leader can make her observations more objective.

8. What is meant by nonverbal communication? How can the team leader put to practical use her knowledge of this method of communication?

9. Observe a worker for several days. Make anecdotal notes of your observations. Criticize each note for completeness and objectivity.

10. If you observe a person performing a procedure incorrectly and you correct her immediately, should you make an anecdotal note of the incident? Give your reasons. How will you be able to determine the progress of this person?

11. Discuss the method or methods you would use to correct a nurses' aide in each of the following situations:
    a. When you observe her taking a glassful of water into the room of a patient who is not allowed to have fluids.
    b. When you observe her removing the weights from a traction apparatus before starting the patient's bath.
    c. When you observe her putting an uncovered hot water bottle at the feet of a patient.
    d. When you overhear her discussing the diagnosis and symptoms of a certain patient with another patient.
    e. When you discover, after she has finished her work, that she failed to clean up an incontinent patient thoroughly.
    f. When, in the course of a report, you discover that she had not given one of the patients an enema that had been ordered.

12. Discuss the statement, "Practice makes perfect."

13. Discuss the various ways in which a team leader may increase the amount of supervision she gives.

14. What is meant by good human relations? What factors will help to improve human relations within the team itself? between team members and patient? between team members and other hospital personnel?

15. Discuss how communication, or the lack of it, affects interpersonal relationships within a family group, within a team, between two teams, within the hospital.

7

HOW TO CONDUCT THE TEAM CONFERENCE

PURPOSES OF THE TEAM CONFERENCE

The conference is the nucleus of team nursing—the center from which all team activities stem. The conference and the resulting plan of nursing care help to differentiate this method of assignment from the functional method. Here you have the opportunity to encourage group dynamics and to cement team spirit. Here also your team members are able to find the answers to their questions concerning the patients, their diseases, and their care. The conference should be helpful and gratifying to you and to each member of your group. The patient benefits because of the consideration given to him as an individual during the conference.

To Plan the Care of the Individual Patient. The emphasis during the discussion is placed on the patient and the nursing care he needs. Any explanation of his disease is incidental and is given only when necessary to help the team to understand the patient's symptoms, behavior, or treatment. For example, the team should be able to give better care to a patient who has hyperthyroidism when they realize that the patient's desire to have her room kept cool, her extreme restlessness, and large appetite are caused by her disease.

When a patient enters the hospital, his doctor is concerned with making a medical diagnosis and developing a plan of therapy. As a nurse, you should also be interested in making a diagnosis, except that your diagnosis is concerned with nursing problems. Your knowledge of the patient's condition and symptoms and how they affect him, combined with your observations and those of your team members, must be used to identify these problems. Like the doctor, you are also interested in developing a plan, except that your plan involves the nursing care the patient needs. With the help of your team, you work out methods of giving this nursing care, including those aspects of treatment that have been delegated by the physician. Your plan may include the modification of specific nursing procedures, the teaching and encouragement the patient needs, and the way of utilizing the services of the other members of the health team and the community. As the problems of the patient change, his care plan must also be changed.

Continuity in the care of the patient is aided by the discussion during the team conference and by the written nursing care plan, which is a record of the care each patient needs and how it should be given. Therefore, you must stress to each person on your team the importance of using the nursing care plans in her work in order to help the patient to recover as quickly as possible.

The emphasis of this conference must always be on evaluation of patient needs and planning patient care. The discussion must be more than a report by each team member about what she did for each patient; nor is this the time to make assignments or to plan the work for the day.

To Coordinate All Available Services. During the conference, your team becomes aware of the different services offered to the patient by the hospital, by other members of the health team, and by other agencies within the community. As they make use of some of these, they may find additional sources of help for their patients. For example, a patient had some complications following a radial mastectomy; however, she insisted on going home to her family even though she had a profuse drainage. Her husband was afraid that she would injure herself by working too hard, since they were financially unable to hire someone to do the housework and care for the children. The help of the local chapter of the American Cancer Society was enlisted to supply dressings. One of the workers there suggested consulting a group of women from a nearby church who helped in times of sickness by going into the home, doing the heavier housework and looking after the children when necessary. The family was happy with the suggestion, so arrangements were made with the women's group. Thus, by making use of one community agency, the team discovered another source of help.

To Promote Team Spirit. As your team members work together, learning more about their patients, and participating in the planning and giving of their care, the spirit of teamwork is stimulated by the feeling of satisfaction, which comes when they are able to do their work well. During the conference, you can also encourage cooperation by constantly stressing the contribution each individual makes toward the work of the team as a whole. No one should be allowed to talk about "my" patients; rather everyone should be encouraged to speak of "our" patients, for, in team nursing, a number of people work together so closely that the team functions as one person.

To Increase the Understanding of the Team. The ability to work together develops only as each person learns more about what good nursing care is and what her role is in providing that care. Your team will acquire more understanding as you supervise them in the performance of their duties. Supervision is also carried on during the team conference. As you observe and listen to the discussion, areas in which the team need more understanding may appear. Some instruction can be given to the entire group during the conference. How to talk with patients, what to say and what not to say, interpretation of hospital policies, the ethics involved in keeping confidential all personal information about the patient — these are only a few topics that may grow out of the discussion of specific problems of a patient.

Team nursing cannot be carried on unless there is a team conference and a written nursing care plan to use as a guide in caring for the patient. Any other method becomes a variation of the functional, assembly-line type of care, which has caused the public to criticize nursing and nurses so harshly.

PLANNING FOR THE CONFERENCE

Some preliminary planning is necessary to keep the conference moving smoothly and to help everyone to benefit by participating in planning the nursing care for their patients.

Planning for Individualized Patient Care. The question sometimes arises concerning the value of having a conference if only two people are on duty and each one is caring for different patients. However, there is no set number of people necessary in order to hold a conference. Remember that one of the important functions of team nursing is the planning of individualized nursing care. Even one person, such as a night nurse working alone without the assistance of a nurses' aide, should have a part in contributing to the plan of care for any patient. For example, she may leave suggestions concerning specific care that will help the patient rest during the night or that will help other nurses care for the patient. This will give the patient a feeling of security as well as providing for continuity of care.

One head nurse noted that a certain patient was always very restless whenever the regular night nurse was off duty. When she questioned this nurse, the head nurse discovered that the patient liked to be prepared for sleep about twelve o'clock. The regular night nurse always planned her work so that she could spend some time with this patient, rubbing his back, fixing his room as he liked it, and following this with a glassful of warm milk and a cheerful goodnight. The patient would then sleep soundly until his early morning treatment. These are little things, yes, but very important to the patient who recognized that the other nurses did not know about this part of his care. The patient thought, perhaps unconsciously, that they did not know about the rest of his care; consequently, he became worried and restless. This aspect of care was recorded on the patient's care plan and when everyone followed the same routine, the patient slept well every night; it made no difference which nurse was on duty.

Selecting the Best Time. A time for the team conference must be selected with the work of the other teams in mind since you cannot leave your patients unattended while your team is having its conference. Select a time which does not conflict with the work of the other personnel; then stick to it everyday. In addition, your team must know where to meet so that each one can arrange her work and be there on time. Soon everyone will accept the conference as part of the day's routine. It is, however, your responsibility to remind them; therefore, post a notice on the station bulletin board, giving the time and the place of the conference along with the name of the patient or patients to be discussed. This information could also be noted on each person's assignment sheet.

The conference does not have to be lengthy. Getting your group together for even 5 or 10 minutes of rapidly moving patient-centered discussion is much better than 20 or 30 minutes of rambling talk. Of course, the more time you have available, the more details you can discuss. However, it is better to start with a short daily conference and increase the time later as you and your team become more adept in using the conference to plan care.

Team nursing can function effectively during the evening and night hours. This means that the team must have a nursing care conference during each shift. Again the choice of the best time will depend upon how ward activities are planned. If the staff changes frequently, the team leader should have the conference during the early part of the shift so that the plans for the care of each particular patient may be used immediately.

Selecting a Patient. Knowing beforehand which patient will be considered is a very important part of planning for the team conference. Ideally, the patient should be chosen the day before the conference, but this may not always be possible. However, this

HOW TO CONDUCT THE TEAM CONFERENCE

information should be available by the time of the team report so that everyone has some time to become acquainted with the patient.

The question of selecting a patient for the conference can be difficult sometimes. Here are some suggestions to consider when making your selection. The patient who has been admitted to the hospital within the last 24 hours needs first consideration. Suppose one has been admitted for diagnosis. Some of the problems that you can readily foresee concern the patient's feelings toward his illness, his fear of the unknown diagnosis, and observations that can be made to help the doctor in making a diagnosis. Perhaps another patient has been admitted to be prepared for surgery during the next few days. Here again some problems may appear to you, for example, the feelings of this patient about the impending surgery and its possible outcome, or the teaching that should be done before surgery. In either case, you need to decide which patient has the more pressing problems. Of course, if you have time, you may wish to consider both patients at the same conference, identifying only the main problem of each patient.

Additional consideration must be given to the fact that a patient's condition is never static. There is always some change and, with that change, some problems may disappear while new ones appear. As team leader, you must review the progress of each patient. Sometimes even though a patient has recently been discussed, a new and serious problem develops, which was unforeseen at the time of the first conference. You may wish to use one conference to review and revise the nursing care plans for a number of patients. If any of your team members report difficulties encountered when giving care to certain patients, the group can discuss and clarify the causes for the difficulties and then develop a satisfactory approach.

Patients who are in the hospital because of a slowly progressive disease, or who have a long convalescence, may be forgotten unless you make it a general rule to periodically evaluate the nursing care needs of these long-term patients. The changes in their conditions may be so indefinite that there seems to be almost none at all. Yet some change always occurs, either emotional or physical, if not both, and with those changes come different problems, which necessitate different approaches.

Frequently, team members will show an interest in a particular patient, not always because of his problems, but because of their interest in his condition or in him as a person. Whenever possible, the team should be allowed to choose the patient or patients they would like to discuss. Their interest will always stimulate more discussion and better planning for individualized care.

Preparation of a Team Leader. You must make a certain amount of personal preparation for the conference. First of all, you must know as much as possible about the patient and his condition from your own personal observation. You may wish to give a part of his care in order to allow yourself time to talk with him; at least, you will need to visit him. In addition, you may want to spend some time in review of the disease and the reasons for the treatment the physican has ordered. However, you will find before long that, as you increase in experience, your need for this preliminary study will decrease, although you must always review in your own mind what you know about the patient's condition, comparing it with what your team members should know.

The possibility of being unable to answer the questions that their team members may ask causes some team leaders to approach the conference with fear and trembling. However, any well-prepared team leader should have no qualms in this respect. There is no person in the world who knows everything or is able to answer every question, and the team members will not expect that much of their leader.

As part of your own preparation, you should plan the points, preferably in writing, that you want to bring out in the discussion.

Illustration

This is the first conference on Mr. Olson, a 42 year old bank cashier, who has a bleeding peptic ulcer. He is receiving antacid and sedative medications between the feedings of a modified Sippy diet.
Questions to be considered:
1. What is a bleeding peptic ulcer? What is the aim of the doctor's treatment?
2. What have you observed about Mr. Olson as a person?
3. Why is he hospitalized? How does he feel about it? What can we tell him?
4. How does he feel about his diet and drugs? What can we tell him?
5. What information do you have about his work, home environment, social life, personal worries, etc.?
6. What are some of his likes and dislikes?

There will be another conference to discuss problems that occur later and to plan for any teaching the patient my need at that time. Your team members may bring out some pertinent observations or have additional questions; however, with this brief outline you can keep the discussion patient-centered and moving smoothly forward.

Preparation of Your Team Members. Team members need to prepare themselves for the conference. You can help by giving them an assignment relative to the patient, although you will not be so crude as to call it an assignment. In this way, you can direct their thinking in various channels toward the search for information they can use in the discussion.

During the team report, while you are explaining the assignments, you may suggest to the team as a whole, but especially to the one who is assigned to care for Mr. Olson, that they observe for answers to such questions as:
1. Does Mr. Olson seem nervous and tense?
2. What topics of conversation did he bring up?
3. Has he been in the hospital before?
4. What questions did he ask about his condition, treatment, etc.?
5. Did he say anything about his work, his home or social life?

In this way, you are laying the foundation for the coming conference so that your team members will have something to contribute to the discussion.

CONDUCTING THE CONFERENCE

Always start the conference on time. Don't wait for the late ones to come for, if you do, they will come later and later each time. When they discover that they are missing something, they will try to be more prompt.

Before starting the discussion, try to make everyone comfortable and at ease. Seating the group in a circle will give the impression of group unity and will encourage each person to participate. Show your interest in each individual and your appreciation for her contribution. Remember that the team conference is an informal discussion by the entire team, not a lecture given by the leader.

Starting the Discussion. You may want to begin with a brief review of the patient's condition. Sometimes the temptation is very strong to spend too much time discussing the disease, especially if it is rare or has been difficult to diagnose. Always remember the background of your team members and make explanations, if they are absolutely necessary, as brief and simple as possible. Include only that information necessary to explain the patient's needs and problems. If the disease is one with which the team is familiar, you may omit this general information in order to provide more time for considering the problems of the patient.

During a later conference, additional information may be given, if the team shows need of it, to increase their understanding of the patient. The team conference is not a ward class. It is not concerned primarily with teaching about the treatment and nursing care of a patient who has a certain disease. It is concerned with developing a satisfactory plan to be used as a guide by those who take care of this particular patient.

Now is the time to begin drawing out the information. There are many ways to get this discussion started, for example you could say:

>"Mr. Olson told me this morning that . . . . Did he indicate this to any of you?"
>
>"Miss A., I noticed that as you took care of Mr. Olson you had no difficulty in getting him to talk. Did he tell you anything about . . . ?"
>
>"According to his chart, he is working at. . . . I wonder if he is working too hard or is worrying about something?"
>
>"I noticed that Mr. Olson made a face when his milk and cream were brought to him. Do you suppose he doesn't like milk?"

Responsibilities of the Conference Leader. Leadership is very important during the team conference, because the kind of nursing care each patient will receive is based upon the care plan developed by the group. When the leadership is used wisely, the team will feel that they are planning the care by themselves. Yet the leader must guide and control her group throughout the entire conference.

KEEP THE DISCUSSION PATIENT-CENTERED. Your main responsibilities are to keep the group thinking about the needs of the specific patient and to keep the discussion "moving forward" toward a solution of his problems. As a rule, you should discourage anyone who tries to bring another patient into the discussion, unless a comparison is being made that will help the group to understand this patient in some specific way. As much as possible, avoid repetition by reminding the group that the information has already been given. Some people find it difficult to speak briefly or to bring out points in a logical order. Sometimes you can help by interrupting with a summarizing statement. If the group begins to digress, bring them back quickly by reminding them of the subject that should be discussed.

ENCOURAGE ALL TEAM MEMBERS TO PARTICIPATE. Throughout the entire conference, you must provide the opportunity and encouragement for making all team members feel free to participate. At no time should one person, including the leader, do most of the talking. You are to act as moderator and guide, using suggestions and questions to help the group to decide how to give care to a particular patient. When presenting a question for the consideration of the group, give them some time for thought. A moment of silence does not mean that you must answer your own question immediately. Throughout the discussion, you need to recognize the abilities of each person and help each one to improve her ability to express her ideas, to understand the patient and his needs, and to plan his care.

Acknowledge each contribution in such a way that the person is encouraged to participate again. It is easy to give this recognition when her contribution has been correct and valuable; however, a problem arises when her information is incorrect or incomplete. Corrections and additions must be made so that everyone will know what is right, yet care must be taken lest the person become discouraged and not try again. You may meet this situation in a number of ways, for example if the information is incomplete, you may say:

> "Do any of you have anything further to add?" or sometimes simply say, "And?"
>
> "Did you think through the entire question?"
>
> "Let me word the question this way," or "Let's approach the problem from this angle." Then rephrase your original question.
>
> "There is more yet. Can any of you think what it might be?"
>
> "I hadn't thought of that, but it's a good idea. However, I had something else in mind."

If the statement is incorrect, either in part or in whole, you may wish to acknowledge the contribution by saying:

> "Most of what you say is correct, but I wonder about . . . ?"
>
> "Do you all agree with that statement?"
>
> "Are you sure that what you are saying is correct?"
>
> "I wonder if you heard the question correctly?"
>
> "I believe that you may have missed the point somewhat. Isn't it true that . . . ?"
>
> "Where did you find your information?"

As a rule, it is wise to avoid asking questions that can be answered by either "Yes" or "No," except when you wish to limit the discussion by a person who talks too much. If you do ask such a question, you may want to follow with the questions, "How?" or "Why?", in order to stimulate more discussion.

UTILIZE ALL OPPORTUNITIES FOR TEACHING. While teaching is not the primary purpose of the team conference, it can be a valuable outgrowth of the discussion, particularly when it concerns methods for improving the nursing care or areas related to ethics or attitudes. You can do this teaching quite often by means of suggestions or leading questions rather than by dogmatic statements. For example, you could say:

"Do you suppose we could . . . ?"
"Would it be wiser to . . . ?"
"Do you mean that . . . ?"
"Is it possible to . . . ?"
"Your suggestion will work, but . . ."
"How do you think the patient would feel about . . . ?"
"How would you feel if you were the patient?"

You must assist your team to recognize the problems in nursing care and to develop suitable methods of solving the problems of each patient. Your team will probably recognize that pain is a problem to a certain patient and may suggest, "Keep the patient comfortable." However, this can be said for many patients. Since the aim of team nursing is to provide *individualized patient care*, you must help your team to decide *how* to keep this particular patient comfortable.

Another area in which teaching opportunities arise is related to the reasons for the emotional reactions manifested by the patient. Perhaps a certain patient is extremely irritable and often critical of everything done for him. During the discussion, reference is made to the fact that "He is an old crab," or "You can't please him no matter what you do." This is your signal that the group needs some teaching to increase their understanding of a specific need or reason for the particular behavior of this patient. When they understand why the patient reacts as he does, you can plan together an approach that will help the patient. Perhaps you decide that this is his way of "getting even" with the hospital routines, which regulate his every move and allow him nothing whatsoever to say. Asking him to choose between two different times for the giving of certain care or consulting him about how he wants his room arranged may be all that is necessary to make him more cheerful and cooperative.

Perhaps at this point something should be said about questions asked by your team members. As a rule, you should always encourage your team to ask questions. This does not mean that you will answer every question. Remember that you cannot allow the discussion to be sidetracked from the patient. You may have to tell the person that a particular question cannot be considered at this time. If a question is asked that you feel the team members, or at least one of them, should be able to answer, hand it back to the group. Make them do a little thinking. On the other hand, a question may arise which is actually beyond the understanding of the group. It is at this point that many team leaders get panicky. Here are some suggestions to help you if you experience this reaction:

    1. Whenever possible, answer the question, using simple terms and not too much detail.

    2. If you don't know the answer, do not try to bluff. Tell

your group frankly that you do not know. You will gain much more respect from your team. Then plan to find the answer. You may ask someone in the group to look up the information, or you may indicate that you will find it and tell them at the next conference. Then keep your promise.

EVALUATE AND SUMMARIZE. You are a listener as your team members bring out their thoughts and observations. You must evaluate all that is said and sift out that which is important for the good of the patient. Your team may not always realize the significance of what the patient said or of what they see. You are the one who will make use of this information. No item is too small to be considered since it may be the final clue needed to determine the nursing care that the patient should have.

RECORD PROBLEMS AND APPROACHES AS EACH IS DECIDED UPON. As the conference progresses, you should record on the nursing care plan those problems and approaches you have helped your team to recognize. Do not try to identify any set number of problems for every patient. One patient may have only one problem, whereas another may have two, and still another may have four or five areas in which plans for specific nursing care must be made. The main thing is to consider the *total* needs of the patient. Then select one or two main problems. It is better to identify and solve one real problem than to look for many problems and offer only superficial suggestions for their solution.

DETERMINE AND RECORD THE AIM OF NURSING CARE. Following the planning of the nursing care, you must help your team to determine the over-all objective or aim of care for the patient. This aim arises from, or is based upon, the needs and approaches already recorded or upon the aim of therapy planned by the doctor. Although general in form, it cannot be made too general. For example, wording the objective this way, "To help the patient get well," is a general aim, which is true for every patient in the hospital. It must be made more specific. The techniques of identifying and wording the problems and plan of care, as well as formulating the aim of care will be found in the next chapter.

USE THE INFORMATION FROM THE NURSING CARE PLAN. The conference and resulting plan of care will benefit the patient only if the information is used. Refer to the care plan when making out assignments and when giving or receiving reports. Use it as a guide when giving nursing care. Show your team how to use the plans. Gradually, you will find everyone depending more and more on them for information concerning how to care for their patients. As a result, the functional approach to nursing care will be eliminated and everyone—patients and workers alike—will be happier and more satisfied.

Close the conference on time even though the group is still interested in further discussion. Under no circumstances allow the conference to "drag" even if the allotted time has not been used. By closing while interest is still high, you are preparing your team for the next conference.

Maintaining Group Control during the Conference. Every group is made up of individuals. If you can control each person and help her to make satisfactory contributions to the general discussion, you will have few problems in controlling the group as a whole. A number of general suggestions have already been made to help you guide the discussion of your team. Here are a few additional suggestions concerning individual and group control:

THE PERSON WHO TALKS TOO MUCH. This individual is always ready to answer at some length any question you may ask. Often she will include unnecessary information. You may use any one of several techniques to control her participation and to give others the opportunity to express their ideas. You may look at your watch, wait for the end of a sentence, then interrupt her and thank her for her contribution; then suggest that you want to hear the opinions of someone else or ask what point is being made. When you ask a question of her, word it so that she needs to answer either "Yes" or "No." Sometimes you will have to ignore her when she indicates that she wishes to talk. This individual may, however, do most of the talking because she actually knows more than the rest of the group; therefore, they rely on her to provide the necessary information. In that case, try to draw out the others first, then use this person to summarize or to give additional information.

THE PERSON WHO TALKS TOO LITTLE. There are usually one or two such people in every group. They may be bored, uninterested, or shy. If possible, determine the reason for their lack of contribution. Find something of interest to the person and ask her to talk about it. If the individual is afraid to speak in front of a group, give her a chance to prepare, by asking her to find out beforehand some specific information about the patient; then ask for her experience or information. Usually it is necessary to call on this person directly. Always thank her for her contribution when she has finished.

PERSONS CARRYING ON A PRIVATE CONVERSATION. Keep the discussion moving fast enough so that everyone will have to listen in order to keep up with the ideas being offered. When you notice a private conversation in progress, pause and let the others listen. You may also ask these people to give their information to the entire group. Another way of breaking in is to ask a direct question of the one who is doing most of the talking.

CONTROLLING AN ANTAGONISTIC GROUP. Occasionally, you may sense a feeling of antagonism within the group during a team conference. If possible, discover the cause. Get the antagonistic persons to talk about their work. If their antagonism is caused by a lack of information or a misunderstanding, try to correct this condition immediately. The group must be able to work together cooperatively if they are to plan good nursing care. Avoid seeming to "push" them. Use those who seem more responsive to help change the feelings of the others. Praise them whenever possible. If you feel that one person is responsible for the attitude of the group as a whole, you may need to have a private conference with her in an effort to clear up her antagonism.

CONTROLLING A PASSIVE GROUP. To encourage participation, discover some point of interest and get passive people to talk about that; however, avoid allowing one or two of the group to do all of the talking. Use more illustrations. Ask simple leading questions. Give additional praise for participation.

CONTROLLING AN ACTIVE GROUP. The group who think quickly and participate readily and actively present a great challenge. Keep ahead of them, moving quickly from point to point. Avoid superficial consideration of the problem under consideration. Use more difficult questions, thus encouraging the group to give more thought to the subject being discussed. Keep the discussion patient-centered.

The conference gives you the opportunity to know your team members better and to weld them into an integrated group capable of working together harmoniously and cooperatively. Your success as a conference leader will enhance your leadership of your team at work.

QUESTIONS ASKED ABOUT THE TEAM CONFERENCE

Why is a conference necessary? The team conference is the only practical means whereby everyone's ideas, observations, and suggestions about the patient and his care can be combined and the best ones selected. When you recognize the wealth of information that the members of your team have about the patients, you will want to make use of it whenever possible. Unless all of you work together toward a common goal, you do not have a team. The leader who "bosses" those who "work for" her does not have a team. The conference helps all your team members to feel that they have a responsibility toward the patient, because they helped in the planning of his care. Unless your group meet together as a team to discuss and plan the nursing care for each patient, you do not have team nursing.

How can I find time for the team conference? This depends upon how strongly you want to hold the conference. If you are really convinced that the conference is necessary to team practice, then you will find the time. Review the day's program, then select a time when there seem to be fewer activities. Most people find that this occurs in the early afternoon or early evening. Now survey the work of the team. Do some scientific thinking, research, problem-solving, or whatever you want to call it, in order to determine where you can reorganize or revise the team's activities to save 10 or 15 minutes a day. Then use that time for your team conference.

How personal can you make the discussion about the patient? A discussion may be as personal as is necessary to help the members of your team understand the patient and why he needs certain care. This is also an excellent time to review the principles of ethics concerning confidential information. I am always amazed at the amount of knowledge that the nurses' aides, and even the housekeeping workers, have about the personal lives of our patients. However, I wonder if we are helping these people to use their information correctly. On the other hand, if a patient requests your help in a confidential matter and you are able to give him the necessary assistance, you would not need to bring this information to the conference because you have already taken care of the problem.

What should be on the conference agenda? The topics you can discuss at the conference will be determined by the needs of your patients and the needs of your team. Usually the needs of the team are based upon, or are outgrowths of, the needs of the patients. Various topics, in addition to the planning of the nursing care for a certain patient or for a number of patients, may include questions the team want answered, difficulties they have encountered in their relationships with patients, difficulties in performing certain procedures or in giving certain aspects of care, or problems in coordinating the work of several individuals, etc.

STUDY QUESTIONS

1. What are the results of the team conference?
2. What methods or suggestions could you use to overcome the resistance of the team members toward spending time in a conference?

HOW TO CONDUCT THE TEAM CONFERENCE

3. What are the best times for holding the team conference?
4. Tell how team nursing, including the holding of the team conference and the making of the nursing care plans, can be practiced throughout the 24 hours in your hospital.
5. What is the difference between the team conference and the conference held at the time of the patient report and explanation of the assignments?
6. Should any member other than the team leader be given the responsibility of leading the conference? Why?
7. Select a patient for a conference. Discuss your own preparation and that of the members of your team.
8. What methods can be used so that every patient assigned to your team will be considered at some team conference and have a nursing care plan?
9. What factors need to be considered when selecting a patient for a conference?
10. Select as many methods as possible that you can use to keep the conference discussion patient-centered.
11. What incidental teaching concerning ethics could be done during the team conference?
12. Discuss each responsibility of the conference leader. What techniques can be used to meet each responsibility?
13. Devise a rating scale for evaluating the effectiveness of the conference leader.
14. Should personal or confidential information about a patient be discussed during the conference? Give reasons for and against. How can you determine what information should be included and what, if any, should not be?
15. Explain briefly and in as simple terms as possible, as you would to a group of nurses' aides, each of the following:
    a. Myocardial infarction
    b. Cheyne-Stokes respiration
    c. Spinogram
    d. Auricular fibrillation
    e. Sympathectomy
    f. Atelectasis
    g. Iodine uptake test
    h. Hydronephrosis
    i. T-tube drainage
    j. Retinal detachment

8

HOW TO MAKE AND TO USE NURSING CARE PLANS

The aim of team nursing is directed toward the improvement of nursing care by utilizing the abilities of a number of people to provide continuous care for the patient, based on his individual needs. The team conference and the resulting nursing care plan are essential in order to achieve this goal.

PURPOSES OF THE NURSING CARE PLAN

To Provide a Guide to Patient-centered Care. One of the main reasons for making a nursing care plan is to provide a guide for patient-centered, rather than job-centered, care. The plan is an outgrowth of discussion, during which every team member focuses her attention on the problems and needs of the patient as an individual and suggests ways for giving the care he needs. The patient is always considered first. His disease is important only to the extent that it affects the physical and emotional aspects of his nursing care.

To Provide a Means of Communication. Another reason for the written nursing care plan is to provide a means of communication

HOW TO MAKE AND TO USE NURSING CARE PLANS

to all personnel. In this way, everyone caring for the patient will receive the benefit of the plan, suggested by the team, and will be better able to carry on a program of continuous individualized care. The written plan is valuable to each worker, especially the professional nurse, as an introduction to the patient and the care given by preceding workers.

To Provide a Guide for Supervising the Team. Since the plan gives information about what nursing care is needed and how it is to be given, it provides the team leader with a guide for her supervision of the team. By using the plan she can make certain that each patient receives the nursing care that is important to him.

To Provide a Basis for Evaluating Patient Care. Because the nursing profession does not yet agree on a specific definition of nursing care, nurses tend to evaluate their care on the basis of proficiency in techniques alone. Yet the team leader should evaluate both the quality and quantity of *nursing* care provided by her team. A well-made nursing care plan defines the care for the individual patient or at least a part of it. By referring to this plan, the team leader can begin her evaluation by asking herself, "How well did we meet the needs of this patient as suggested in the nursing care plan?"

ESSENTIAL PARTS OF A PATIENT CARE PLAN

Today nursing care is defined as the action that the nurse takes in fulfilling her primary function. Yet the nurse also gives care which is prescribed by the doctor or dictated by hospital policy; therefore, to differentiate between this delegated care and nursing care, the term *patient care* is used here to describe *all* care for which the nurse is responsible. Patient care includes three aspects: the medical care which is prescribed by the doctor but delegated to others, general care which may be prescribed by the doctor or set by hospital policy, and nursing care which the nurse, functioning as an independent practitioner, determines is necessary to help her patient.

Delegated Medical Care. The physician's primary responsibility is diagnosis and treatment of illness; however, he delegates some of the diagnostic and therapeutic techniques. This delegated medical care is commonly recorded on the Kardex under the heading of medications and treatments. Those aspects of patient care for which the nurse is not responsible, except to see that they are done, e.g., laboratory tests or physiotherapy, may be listed separately under other headings.

General Patient Care. Food and fluid requirements, amount of physical activity, and personal hygiene measures may be determined by the patient's illness and the doctor's plan of therapy; however, the time that meals are served or the bath given is often a matter of hospital policy. These aspects of patient care are usually recorded under the heading of general care or general nursing measures.

Nursing Care. Each patient responds in a different way to illness and its treatment, to his social environment and economic state. He may not even show the same response consistently day after day. He has his own peculiar likes, dislikes, worries, and fears.

Although the nurse works within the dictates of the plan of medical care and of established hospital policy, she must identify the nursing needs of her patient and determine how to meet them. In other words, she makes a nursing diagnosis and prescribes the nursing care needed to solve each nursing problem.

Nursing care may be related to some part of the delegated medical care, e.g., determining what is causing a patient's discomfort and what should be done to make him more comfortable. Nursing care is also needed to adapt a general hospital routine to fit the needs of the individual patient, e.g., selecting the best time and method to make him comfortable for sleep. Nursing care is that help given to the patient to assist him through his illness by minimizing as much as possible the source of his tensions, e.g., cleansing his mouth before a meal to make the food taste better, thereby encouraging him to eat.

In order to give nursing care the team leader and her team must know as much as possible about the patient. In some cases, the nurse will need to use all her knowledge and skill to determine what the patient wants or needs and how to take care of him. In other cases, planning and giving nursing care may be quite simple. Always the team leader and her team members work together in giving this care.

THE AIM OF NURSING CARE. The aim indicates, in general terms, what the team hopes to accomplish for the patient, or what they can help him to accomplish for himself. It is related to the nursing problems that the team leader and her team have identified and must also take into account the aim of medical therapy.

The patient's diagnosis, religion, marital status, age, etc., are usually written somewhere on the record of the patient care plan. While this information is not directly a part of the plan, it is important to the team because it provides background material that will help them to understand the patient better.

WHEN AND HOW TO BEGIN THE NURSING CARE PLAN

Begin When the Patient Is Admitted. The nursing care plan should be started when the patient enters the hospital. As team leader you will probably have the responsibility for admitting the patient and taking care of the first orders. Although you may delegate part of this routine to someone else, you will need to visit the patient and make your own observations.

Some hospitals are including in the admission routine the use of a structured interview or a nursing admission interview form which becomes part of the patient's record. When the team leader visits the patient during the admission period, she uses this interview method to get enough information in order to start planning individual care. The purpose of this interview is to get to know the patient. The form may list various questions such as the following:

1. Have you been in a hospital before? When? Why?
2. What makes you feel comfortable when you are sick?
3. Are you on any special medication?
4. Do you have any allergies?
5. Do you have any special likes or dislikes about food?
6. Do you have any difficulty sleeping?
7. Do you have any difficulty in bowel elimination? In elimination of urine?
8. Do you want any restriction on visitors?

These questions should suggest others that could be asked. The questions should be planned according to the age and condition of the patient; e.g., the nurse could ask the parents of a small child about special words he uses to express his wants, or about the schedule of activities he is used to at home.

As the nurse talks with the patient, she should observe his appearance, facial expression, speech, and behavior. When she has completed the interview and received reports from anyone else who has been with the patient, she is ready to begin the nursing care plan for the patient.

How To Start the Care Plan. This initial plan is based on the treatment instituted by the doctor and upon any information obtained by you or any other person who helped with the admission of the patient. Perhaps you observe that the patient is hard of hearing or a relative tells you that the patient has been incontinent at home. Write the problem or problems on the nursing care plan along with your suggestions for solving them. If the patient has a hearing aid or can read lips, note it on the plan. If you foresee the possibility of bedsores because of the incontinence, plan now to prevent them. If the doctor ordered the insertion of an indwelling catheter, the incontinence is no longer a nursing problem. Instead, you foresee the possibility of other problems occurring, such as keeping the catheter working properly or minimizing urethral irritation. Perhaps when you give the first dose of medicine, the patient informs you that he cannot swallow pills; here is another problem. So you record the appropriate approach on the care plan or on the medication card, indicating that the tablets must be crushed. You have made a good start already toward individualizing the care of this patient. During these initial observations, you should look for evidence of fear or apprehension in the patient toward his hospitalization, evidence of loss of sight, or any language difficulties. Record what the patient states to be his likes and dislikes, or what he is allergic to. With practice you and your team will find many other areas of information that can easily be included within this period of admitting the patient and starting his treatment. This initial plan may also include the teaching needs of the patient. For example, he should be taught about the tests and examinations ordered for him or about the turning and breathing exercises he must do after surgery.

The listing of any definite problems you see at this time is just as important as the listing of the medications and treatments ordered by the doctor if you are to provide total care of this patient. Later, after your team has become acquainted with the patient, you will evaluate his care at a team conference.

HOW TO PLAN INDIVIDUAL NURSING CARE

Perhaps a word should be said first about what should and should not be included in the plan. In general, the plan should include:
1. Problems concerning the giving of delegated medical care.
2. Problems which affect the method of doing any nursing technique or the carrying out of any responsibility delegated by the doctor.
3. Problems concerning information to be given to the patient or to his relatives.
4. Problems which affect the interpersonal relationships between patient and worker.
5. Problems concerning the patient's response to his environment, his illness, and his inability to care for himself.
6. Suggestions for approaches to the problems, developed specifically for the individual patient.

HOW TO MAKE AND TO USE NURSING CARE PLANS 137

In general the plan should not include:
1. Confidential information about the patient.
2. Suggestions for approaches which are repetitions of hospital routines or of doctor's orders.

How To Identify Needs and Problems of Nursing Care. Needs and problems are not identical, although one grows out of, or is related to, the other. Needs are concerned with the processes necessary for life and with the person's response to his environment. A problem arises when a conflict occurs between one or more of these needs, either because of the effect of disease on the body or because the patient uses an unacceptable way to fulfill a need. For example, the body needs water if it is to carry on its life processes. What happens if the patient is nauseated and refuses all food and fluids; if he is willing to drink but is unable to do so because of mouth surgery; or if he is limited in his fluid intake but insists on drinking too much? In each case, the need and the problem involve the fluid intake of the patient; however, in each situation, the cause of the problem is different. Therefore, the solution must be specific for the cause and thus individualized for the patient.

Outlines I, II, and III, on pages 146, 147, and 148, respectively, give some suggestions to help in the identification of patient needs and nursing problems. Outline I lists some of the factors related to the needs of any individual. You will need to apply your knowledge concerning the patient's condition to know how the disease affects him emotionally and physically, how his response to his environment will change because of this disease, how the disease is treated, and how this treatment may affect the patient. You may wish to ask yourself such questions as:
1. How does this patient's disease modify his normal expression of, or his ability to fulfill, each need?
2. How does the treatment ordered for this patient affect each need?
3. How does the patient "feel" about his disease?
4. How much does the patient know about his condition? How much can he learn?
5. What nursing problems arise because of the effect of the disease on the various needs of the patient?

Illustration A

Mary has just been diagnosed as a diabetic. She knows that her aunt had diabetes and believes that this disease caused her aunt's death a few years after the diagnosis was made. To help this patient, you may consider either her emotional needs or her physical needs first. Mary is afraid because she does not know much about her condition or how to care for herself. She believes the prognosis is hopeless; therefore, she is ready to give up without trying to help herself in any way. You realize immediately that Mary has problems because of her response to the disease. Also her response will influence some of the social and economic aspects of her everyday life. With increased understanding of her condition and of how it can be controlled, some of these problems will be solved.

Considering her physical needs, you can readily see that, since diabetes mellitus is a disturbance of metabolism, the intake and utilization of food, water, and oxygen are affected. The amount of exercise and rest also affect the utilization of these substances. Elimination of body wastes from the lungs and kidneys may also be changed. As you plan Mary's nursing care, you must keep all these changes in mind.

The regulation of the disease and the prevention of complications, such as infection, are important. Therefore, you must give special attention to Mary's environment in order to prevent injury and promote cleanliness. As you plan, you must keep in mind that Mary's main problem seems to be her lack of understanding about the disease and how to live with it; therefore, you need to plan your approach to this patient in relation to what she knows and feels and what she needs to know.

It is at this point that team discussion and planning of this patient's care are necessary. You have done the preliminary thinking, helped undoubtedly by the observations and reports of your team members. You have also identified the main problem, and you may have some ideas concerning appropriate methods of helping the patient. You will not, however, be able, nor should you try, to give all the care that Mary needs. The conference gives your team the opportunity to learn what good nursing care for Mary should include and to plan how everyone may work together in giving that care. The written nursing care plan, which you make as a result of the group discussion and cooperative planning, will serve as a guide in giving and evaluating her care.

In this particular case, the aim of care is related to helping Mary learn about her disease and how to live with it since all of her problems seem to stem from her lack of knowledge and understanding.

Illustration B

The needs and problems of the patient may not always be so readily apparent. For example, Jim Doe is scheduled for an appen-

HOW TO MAKE AND TO USE NURSING CARE PLANS

dectomy because of recurrent appendicitis. He shows no signs of apprehension about his surgery and quickly understands your explanations concerning hospital routines and what will be done for him. After surgery he is cooperative and starts an uneventful convalescence, giving no indication of having any problems. One day as you visit him, he makes several requests, indicating some of his likes and dislikes about his food and care. Make a note of these on his care plan and bring them to the attention of your team. Were these important problems? Not so far as helping in his recovery, but the patient's likes and dislikes are always important to him. Complying with these requests is certainly one way of individualizing his nursing care and is very important in the establishment of good public relations.

How To Identify Needs and Problems Related to Delegated Medical Care and General Care. The responsibilities delegated by the physician to the nurse cannot be ignored when planning the care of the patient. Every nurse is familiar with the five *rights* to be observed when giving medications—the right drug in the right amount to the right patient at the right time and in the right way. Every step of the procedure is based on one or more of these rights. However, these five rights are concerned with technique only and do not indicate the individual nursing care needs of a patient who is receiving a particular drug. Outline II on page 147 offers some suggestions to use in determining problems related to the giving of medications to the patient. The approach to these problems may be recorded either on the medication card or on the nursing care plan or in both places.

Nursing techniques are based upon the principles of safety and comfort for the patient, teaching of the patient, and good workmanship by the nurse. If you are to give individualized nursing care, you cannot perform a nursing technique in exactly the same way for every patient. The principles remain the same, but the method may vary according to the condition, treatment, and needs of each patient. Outline III on page 148 contains some suggestions to use in determining problems involving nursing techniques.

How To Develop Solutions to Nursing Problems. A well-made plan should enable a worker who has never cared for the patient to become acquainted with him and his background and with the way his care has been and should be given. When this plan is used, the patient is no longer a stranger to her, and then the worker has more self-confidence when she approaches him. She already knows something about his likes and dislikes and how to satisfy him.

Here are some illustrations showing how solutions should *not* be worded. In each case, the approach is nonspecific or lacks information concerning the proper methods to be used to meet the special problem of the patient.

PROBLEM	APPROACH
Pain	Keep the patient comfortable or give hypo p.r.n.
Indwelling catheter	Irrigate catheter b.i.d.
Patient is apprehensive	Reassure patient.
Bedsores	Turn patient frequently.
Force fluids	Offer patient water frequently and in small amounts.

Such approaches show little thought for the patient as an individual and give little help to the worker who must care for him. Go back to the outlines containing suggestions for methods of individualizing patient care. Ask yourself the following questions about the problems you have identified:

Is there anything I can do to make the patient more comfortable? Does a back rub help to relieve the pain? Does changing position help? If so, what positions are best?

What makes the indwelling catheter a problem—irritation, malposition, constant plugging? What can I do to relieve or minimize the cause?

Why is the patient apprehensive? What do I mean by "reassure the patient?"

Are there any special techniques to use when turning the patient? Is there any special position that would help to prevent bedsores? How often is frequently?

Why is it necessary to force fluids? How can I encourage the patient to cooperate? Can the patient have anything other than water? If so, what does he like? Again, how often is frequently? How much is a "small amount" for this patient?

The question is sometimes asked whether the doctor must be informed of nursing problems and must agree to the proposed solutions. The aims of the health team, of which both doctor and nurse are members, are to aid in the recovery of the patient and to return him to his home and community where he may function to the limit of his ability. As members of this health team the doctor and nurse cannot afford to function as separate entities. Any problem affecting the patient is the concern of both, and the aim of nursing care cannot be separated from the aim of medical treatment. There must always be communication between doctor and nurse.

Whether the doctor must approve the solutions to the patient's problems as proposed by the team will depend upon two factors. First, it will depend on whether the approach is merely a modification of an accepted hospital policy or nursing procedure or whether it involves some aspect of the medical treatment instituted by the doctor. Secondly, it will depend on the amount of rapport existing between the doctor and nurse and the confidence he has in her use of good judgment.

Suppose the problem involves helping the patient to increase his fluid intake. Perhaps the first approach would be to find out what fluids this patient particularly likes and, therefore, would drink more readily. The problem of adequate fluid intake certainly should be called to the attention of the doctor; however, the nurse's approach at this point does not need his approval. After the team finds out what the patient likes, their solution to the problem may be changed to the provision of those fluids which he prefers. Since this is probably accepted hospital procedure, it does not need to be approved by the doctor, although the nurse will undoubtedly want to keep him informed. On the other hand, if the team finds out that the patient likes some fluids contraindicated by the medical treatment, the doctor must decide whether to change his treatment; therefore, the proposed solution is brought to the doctor's attention and must receive his approval before it can be used.

How To Determine the Objectives of Nursing Care. The aim of nursing care is found in the needs and problems of the patient and may be related either to his inability, because of some problem, to satisfy one or more of his basic needs or to the aim of medical treatment instituted by the doctor. The statement of the objective must be specific to the patient and cannot be merely a repetition of a general aim of care for every patient. For example, the aims, "keep the patient comfortable" and "help the patient learn to care for himself" or "to recover without complications," are valid for every patient in the hospital. The objective must be related to that which the team hopes to accomplish as they care for each particular person. "Keep the patient comfortable" would be an acceptable objective of nursing care only if he is suffering from intractable pain and if the main aim of medical therapy is the alleviation of that pain.

There is no need to list an objective of care for every problem. Rather the objective should be worded in such a way that the most important problem or problems are indicated. For example, "help the patient adjust to his loss of vision" and "help the patient to accept his colostomy and learn how to care for it" indicate the areas where major problems exist for these patients and what the team hopes to accomplish through their approach to each problem.

Planning patient-centered care is not easy but, with practice, you and your team will become better able to consider each patient as an individual, to define his problems and to determine the best way to meet those problems. The quality of nursing care resulting from this kind of planning is a constant source of satisfaction to you and your team, as well as to your patients. In addition, it provides a challenge to improve your knowledge and understanding as you care for each new patient.

HOW TO KEEP NURSING CARE PLANS UP TO DATE

Every professional nurse is responsible for initiating the nursing care plan and for keeping it up-to-date. This includes the head nurse and every staff nurse, whether or not she is a team leader. Any nursing care plan, if it is to be effective, must contain information concerning the care the patient needs at the present time. This present care will also include the foreseeing of future problems and trying to prevent them. Anything that is not related to the patient's present care should be removed from the care plan. Some problems will be solved and new ones will appear because the patient's condition is always changing. Even the long-term patient will present new problems, since, even though they may be barely discernible, physical and emotional changes occur in response to confinement and disability.

Daily team conferences, keeping the care plans up to date and using them constantly, are the prerequisites for effective team action. Current information is necessary if the plan of care is to be of any value to you or to your team. You must find the times when it is most convenient for you to bring the information up to date.

During Rounds to Visit Your Patients. As you visit each of your patients, you may receive information, either from what you see or from what the patient tells you, indicating that a change in his plan of care is necessary. If the change is slight, you can make the adjustment immediately. Perhaps a patient requests that his leg be placed in a certain position when he is sitting in a chair. If that position is not contraindicated, note the patient's request on his care-plan immediately. If for any reason his request cannot be granted, you must take care of the problem at once by giving him sufficient information for him to understand why it is impossible to do as he has requested.

When the Kardex and Patient's Chart Are Checked. The Kardex and each patient's chart are checked at regular intervals to insure that no information is omitted. Usually this is part of the administrative responsibility of the head nurse; however, she may at this time find areas in the care plan which should be changed or have suggestions concerning additional care for the patient. This is especially true if the doctor has changed his plan of treatment. If part of your responsibility involves taking care of the doctor's orders for your patients, remember that it is just as important to check the special problems of the patient as it is to check the plan for his treatments.

When a Report Is Given. One of the most common times for bringing the care plan up to date is at the time of a report. Usually when one shift reports to the next is the time when the professional nurse who does not work with a team offers her suggestions concerning the nursing care she feels the patient needs. She may also report her observations concerning the effectiveness of the various approaches being used. In this way, the private duty nurse or the night nurse is made to feel that she is a contributing member of the team even though she may not actually work with it.

During any report, the entire plan should be noted, not just that part concerned with the doctor's orders. For example, if, during a report about a patient, you note that the indwelling catheter about which there was a problem has been taken out, the notations must be removed from both places in the patient care plan. On the other hand, if you foresee that the removal of the catheter may cause new problems, perhaps that of incontinence or of insuring that the patient is voiding in adequate amounts, this new problem should be noted on the plan at this time, as well as your suggested approach. This new information is then included in your reports to your team and to your head nurse.

At the Team Conference. Although you may make changes in the plan of care whenever you find it necessary, nothing can take the place of the team conference for complete evaluation and planning by the entire group. This is the time for a complete review of the patient's care to insure that all parts of the plan are usable and that nothing has been omitted.

HOW TO USE THE NURSING CARE PLANS

Nursing care plans will be used when the team finds that these plans help them in their work. The more help they receive from the conferences and the written plans, the more they will want them and use them. Your main aim should then be to help the team discover the value of the nursing care plans.

Use the Plans as a Guide for Making Assignments. Coordinate the abilities of the various members of your team with the care your patients need. When discussing the assignment with the worker, refer to the entire plan of care and call her attention to those aspects for which she is responsible.

Refer to the Entire Plan during Every Report Period. Use it as a guide to insure that no part of the patient's care will be, or has been, omitted. You always check to make sure that all treatments and medications have been given; it is just as important to check to make sure that the patient's problems have been recognized and that some attempt has been made to solve them. You try to find out how the patient responded to a treatment or to a drug; it is just as important to find out how the patient reacted to the care given because of his needs and problems. As you get this information, you can evaluate better the effectiveness of the nursing care given by your team.

Use the Plan To Orient Team Members Following Vacation or Days Off. The up-to-date care plan is valuable to show the progress of the patient as well as to indicate present nursing care. By reviewing the care plans, the worker's memory is refreshed concerning those patients she has cared for previously, and she receives an introduction to any new patients and the care that they need.

Use It as a Guide in Supervising and Evaluating the Work of Your Team. The care plan gives you the information concerning the activities you should observe. Since, in your supervision, you are concerned with helping and directing your team, you will need to refer to the nursing care plan to determine what care should be given and whether it is being given correctly.

The nursing care plan is a guide to the care *currently* being given to the patient and cannot take the place of the patient's chart, which is a record of the care that *has been* given. The care plan helps to insure the continuity of safe individualized nursing care around the clock. If the patient is transferred to another section of the hospital, the nursing care plan should be transferred along with his chart. The history of the nursing problems of the patient and how they are being met is just as important for helping everyone to understand the patient and his progress as the medical history and treatment.

If the care plan is used in these ways, it will give the team concrete goals toward which to strive in their work, thus stimulating a feeling of unity and satisfaction within the group.

QUESTIONS ASKED ABOUT NURSING CARE PLANS

How can I convince the nursing personnel of the usefulness and importance of the care plans? The nursing care plan can be just as useful as you want it to be. The personnel will more readily see its value if the plan is carefully thought out and made individual for the patient. Then the plan will help them in their work. Refer to the plan whenever you talk about the patient. Use it in planning your work and when you help your team to plan their

HOW TO MAKE AND TO USE NURSING CARE PLANS

work. Refer to it again to determine if their work has been done properly. When the members of your team see you using the plans continuously, they will use them too.

How can you make out the nursing care plan when you don't have time to talk to the patient? It is impossible to plan the nursing care for the individual unless you are acquainted with him. I believe there are two aspects of this problem that you should consider. First, are you sure that you can't find time to talk *with* the patient? I am sure that as a team leader you must come to his bedside several times during the day; otherwise, you are not assuming your responsibilities as team leader. The problem then becomes one of making the best use of these few minutes, to talk *with*, not *to*, your patient, getting him to talk about himself. You should never allow yourself to become so busy that you do not see or hear the patient as you give him his medicine, put on his hot packs, irrigate his catheter, change his dressings, or make your rounds.

The second aspect of this problem is directly related to one of the reasons for having a team conference. Knowing that you do not have as much time as you would like to become acquainted with the patient, you then must rely upon the eyes and ears of your team members. You need to become skillful in questioning them so that they will relate as many details as possible about the patients. As conference leader, you have the great responsibility, first, of collecting all the information the team members may have; and secondly, of determining the importance of their information in relation to the care the patient needs.

How can the nursing care plan be made more individual for each patient? In order to make the plan individual you must know as much as possible about your patient—his disease and how it affects him, his treatment, his likes and dislikes, his home and family, his worries, and so on. After you have obtained all this information, try to answer some questions about the patient and his care; for example, what care does he need and how and when should it be given?

Where should the nursing care plans be kept? Since the plan for nursing care is only one part of the patient care plan, it must be kept with the rest of the plan, i.e., in the Kardex. Realizing that the Kardex is used frequently, you will need to discuss the information about the nursing care plan at the same time that you discuss the medical care responsibilities (treatments and medications) delegated to you by the physician.

Should all team members read the nursing care plan? Absolutely. If each member of the team is to contribute to the total care of the patient, she must know what and how to do it. Certainly, the nursing care plan should not be the jealously guarded secret of just a few.

STUDY QUESTIONS

1. Select two patients. Applying the suggestions listed in Outlines I, II, and III, below and on pages 147 and 148, individualize every aspect of their care. Be sure to consider all their needs in relation to their disease conditions. Then make a nursing care plan for each patient.
2. While you admit a patient, obtain as much information as you can. Start a care plan for this patient.
3. What are the various reasons for having a written nursing care plan?
4. What are the essential parts of a patient care plan? Discuss the ways in which information can be obtained for each part of the plan.
5. List the times and the methods that can be used on your sections to keep the nursing care plans up to date.
6. Select a number of patients and evaluate their care plans. How much individualized care is indicated? What approaches seem good? Why? Which approaches could be improved? How? Is the aim of nursing care consistent with the problems of the patient or with the plan of therapy ordered by the doctor?
7. Make out an assignment for your team. Indicate how the nursing care plan, especially the part concerned with the special problems of the patient, was used in planning these assignments.
8. Discuss the ways in which greater use can be made of the nursing care plans.

OUTLINE I

Areas To Consider When Determining Special Needs and Problems of the Patient

Physical needs include:
- oxygen, water, food — depending on
  - adequate intake
  - normal digestion
  - normal absorption
  - normal metabolism
- elimination from the
  - skin
  - lungs
  - bowels
  - kidneys
- exercise and rest
- sex

Spiritual and emotional needs involve:
- fear
- anger
- love
- security
- self-worth
- self-expression, etc.

Environmental needs involve:
- warmth
- light
- external stimuli
- safety measures
- cleanliness
- general comfort and welfare measures

Socioeconomic aspects include:
- age
- status in family and community
- religion
- nationality
- economic status, etc.

Therapeutic and rehabilitative needs involve:
- diagnosis of disease
- treatment of disease
- relief of symptoms
- prevention of complications
- teaching self-care
- patient's return to society as a contributing member

Patient teaching needs are found in the needs and problems in any of the above areas in which the patient should increase his understanding, either of his condition and his progress or of himself as a person.

HOW TO MAKE AND TO USE NURSING CARE PLANS

OUTLINE II

Areas To Consider When Determining Nursing Care Necessary with a Particular Drug
- A. How is this drug to be administered?
    1. What are the special methods of preparation of this drug for administration due to its physical and chemical characteristics or to the preference of the patient.
       Example 1: Disguise taste by mixing with fruit juice.
       Example 2: Crush tablet and mix with water.
    2. What special nursing measures should be performed *before* giving the drug?
       Example: Count pulse before giving drug.
    3. What special nursing measures should be performed *during* the administration of the drug?
       Example 1: Give slowly deep into the muscle.
       Example 2: Give through a straw — must not come into contact with teeth.
    4. What special nursing measures or precautions must be used *after* administration of the drug?
       Example: No water allowed after taking drug.
- B. Why does the patient need this drug? What signs and symptoms must be watched for to determine a *satisfactory* response to this drug? A drug may have a number of actions depending upon the pharmacological action, the dosage, the site of administration, and the condition of the patient. Determine what action the doctor expects.
       Example 1: Codeine may be given to control cough or to relieve pain.
       Example 2: Atropine may be given to dry up secretions or to cause relaxation of smooth muscle spasm.
  A satisfactory response to the expected action of this drug is indicated by certain signs and symptoms. The observation for their presence or absence is important nursing care.
- C. What are the most common reactions due to sensitivity, idiosyncrasy, and/or toxicity caused by this drug?
    1. Symptoms of reactions due to sensitivity and idiosyncrasy may not be related to the usual actions of the drug. The nurse must know the common reactions and be alert for those symptoms.
       Example: Penicillin may cause skin rash.
    2. Toxic reactions are frequently related to an overstimulation or overdepression of a certain part of the body beyond that expected as a usual action of the drug. Observe for these signs and symptoms.
       Example 1: Extreme slowness of respiration following the administration of morphine.
       Example 2: Diarrhea occurring with the use of antibiotics.
- D. What nursing measures not directly related to the actual administration or observation of the reactions to this drug can be used to aid the patient in obtaining the desired action or to prevent complications?
    1. Physical and environmental.
       Example 1: With a sleeping pill, use all methods necessary to help patient to relax and get comfortable.
       Example 2: With the administration of aspirin to reduce fever, keep the patient dry and out of drafts to prevent chilling when sweating occurs.
    2. Emotional.
       Example 1: How can the nurse explain to the patient
          a. What the drug is given for?
          b. What he should do because he is receiving it?
       Example 2: The nurse must recognize the psychological effects of color, taste, method of administration, etc.

OUTLINE III

Areas To Consider When Determining Special Needs and Problems of the Patient Treatment or General Nursing Care

    A. Why did the doctor order this treatment for the patient?
        1. What signs and symptoms indicate a satisfactory response to the treatment?
            Example: Mouth and lips less dry and cracked after special oral hygiene.
        2. What would indicate an unsatisfactory response?
            Example: Distention and abdominal pain following an enema.
    B. Physical aspects
        1. What steps of this procedure will be affected by the physical condition of this patient?
            Example 1: Application of hot packs to treat an infected toe of an elderly patient.
            Example 2: Giving and removing a bedpan from an emaciated patient with fragile skin.
        2. How can I make the necessary adaptations and still observe the basic principles of the procedure?
    C. Emotional aspects
        1. How does the patient feel about this treatment?
        2. What explanation can be given to increase his understanding and gain more cooperation?
        3. How can I perform the procedure and still observe the precautions necessary because of the patient's emotional response?
            Example: Application of dermatologic packs to the groin of a very modest patient.

AM I A GOOD TEAM LEADER?

Answer each question by placing a check in the column that you believe best describes your performance.

		1 ALWAYS	2 OFTEN	3 RARELY
1.	Do I believe that team nursing will work?			
2.	Is my work a good example to others?			
3.	Am I enthusiastic about my work?			
4.	Do I try to learn as much as possible about every part of my job?			
5.	Am I able to control my temper?			
6.	Do I think before I speak?			
7.	Do I admit it when I am wrong?			
8.	Do I try to understand the other person's viewpoint?			
9.	Do I feel that each team member is important in caring for the patient?			
10.	Am I able to plan ahead?			
11.	Am I systematic about doing my own work?			
12.	Do I show my confidence in my team?			

HOW TO MAKE AND TO USE NURSING CARE PLANS

13. Do I consider both the worker and the patient when I plan the assignments?
14. Do I give a complete report to every team member?
15. Do I ask more often than I command?
16. Does my team voluntarily seek my advice?
17. Do I check to determine that all assignments have been completed properly?
18. Do I try to be objective in evaluating the work of others?
19. Do I try to find out all the facts before I draw my conclusion?
20. Do I offer praise often?
21. Do I inform my team members of their progress?
22. Do I try to help each member of my team improve?
23. Do I encourage discussion during the team conference?
24. Do I keep the nursing care plans up to date?
25. Do I use the nursing care plans?

Each check in column 1 gives you 4 points, column 2 gives you 2 points, column 3 no points. Total your score.

A score of

92 and over — Congratulations on your excellent leadership!
82 to 91 — Satisfactory, but some improvement is needed.
Below 82 — Start planning at once ways to increase your skills in leadership.

PART THREE BIBLIOGRAPHY

Books

Byrne, Brandon: *Three Weeks to a Better Memory.* John C. Winston Company, Philadelphia, 1952.
Cooper, Joseph D.: *How to Get More Done in Less Time.* Doubleday & Company, Inc. Garden City, N.Y., 1962.
Creighton, Helen: *The Law Every Nurse Should Know.* W. B. Saunders Company, Philadelphia, 1957.
Lambertsen, Eleanor: *Nursing Team — Organization and Functioning.* Published for the Division of Nursing Education, Bureau of Publications, Teacher's College, Columbia University, New York, 1953.
Leadership on the Job — Guides to Good Supervision. Edited by the staff of Supervisory Management. Published by the American Management Association, New York, 1957.
Lesnik, Milton J., and Anderson, Bernice E.: *Nursing Practice and the Law.* J. B. Lippincott Company, Philadelphia, 1962.
Murphy, Dennis: *Better Business Communication.* McGraw-Hill Book Company, Inc., New York, 1957.
Newcomb, Dorothy Perkins: *The Team Plan, A Manual for Nursing Service Administrators.* G. P. Putnam's Sons, Inc., New York, 1953.
Osborn, Alex F.: *Applied Imagination.* Charles Scribner's Sons, New York, 1957.
Perrodin, Cecilia M.: *Supervision of Nursing Service Personnel.* The Macmillan Company, New York, 1957.
Pieper, Frank: *Modular Management and Human Leadership.* Methods Press, Minneapolis, 1958.

Journals

Brackett, Mary E., and Fogt, Joan R.: *Is Comprehensive Nursing Care a Realistic Goal?* Nurs. Outlook, 9:7:402, July, 1961.
Bratton, Jimmie K.: *A Definition of Comprehensive Nursing Care.* Nurs. Outlook, 9:8:481, Aug., 1961.
Brooks, Ethel A.: *Team Nursing*—1961. Am. J. Nursing, 61:4:87, April, 1961.
Chambers, Wilda: *Nursing Diagnosis.* Am. J. Nursing, 62:11:102, Nov., 1962.
Coletti, Angela C.: *The Head Nurse Is a Manager.* Hospital Progress, 41:3:100, March, 1960.
Corona, Dorothy F., and Black, Eunice E.: *One Hospital's Approach to Team Nursing.* Nurs. Outlook, 11:7:506, July, 1963.
Creighton, Helen: *The Liability of the Surgical Nurse.* Hospital Management, 99:1:46, Jan., 1965.
Donovan, Helen M.: *Determining Priorities of Nursing Care.* Nurs. Outlook, 11:1:44, Jan., 1963.
Elizabeth, Sister Regina: *Team Nursing Revised.* Hospital Progress, 45(7):112, July, 1964.
Fogt, Joan: *Team Nursing: Concepts and Procedures.* Hospital Progress, 45(2):65, Feb., 1964.
Fogt, Joan: *Team Nursing: Inservice Education for the Team Leader.* Hospital Progress, 45(4):31, April, 1964.
Fogt, Joan: *Team Nursing: The Team Leader.* Hospital Progress, 45(3):104, March, 1964.
Geister, Janet M.: *Public Relations Begin at the Bedside.* Am. J. Nursing, 50:8:463, Aug., 1950.
Gerard, Richard W.: *The Importance of Communication.* Hospital Management, 89:5:73, May, 1960.
Gladieux, Bernard N.: *Organization—Planned and Defined.* Hospital Progress, 41:1:53, Jan., 1960.
Gordon, Phoebe: *Evaluation, A Tool of Nursing Service.* Am. J. Nursing, 60:3:364, March, 1960.
Gozzi, Ethel Kontz: *We Plan Ahead What To Ask.* Nurs. Outlook, 13:6:30, June, 1965.
Gregg, Dorothy: *Reassurance.* Am. J. Nursing, 55:2:171, Feb., 1955.
Hay, Stella I., and Anderson, Helen C.: *Are Nurses Meeting Patients' Needs?* Am. J. Nursing, 63:12:97, Dec., 1963.
Henderson, Virginia: *The Nature of Nursing.* Am. J. Nursing, 64:8:62, Aug., 1964.
Hershey, Nathan: *Doctrine of Respondeat Superior.* Am. J. Nursing, 62:4:78, April, 1962.
Hershey, Nathan: *A Nurse's Liability for Negligence in Supervision.* Am. J. Nursing, 62:5:115, May, 1962.
Horty, John S.: *How Hospital Law Is Changing.* Modern Hospital, 96:1:71, Jan., 1961.
How To Plan Work. Management course for Air Force supervisors. Air Force Pamphlet No. 50-2-10, United States Government Printing Office, Washington, D.C., June, 1955.
How To Direct and Coordinate Work. Management course for Air Force supervisors. Air Force Pamphlet No. 50-2-11, United States Government Printing Office, Washington, D.C., June, 1955.
How To Instruct the Worker. Management course for Air Force supervisors. Air Force Pamphlet No. 50-2-16, United States Govefnment Printing Office, Washington, D.C., June, 1955.
How To Apply Techniques of Good Human Relations. Management course for Air Force supervisors. Air Force Pamphlet No. 50-2-19, United States Government Printing Office, Washington, D.C., June, 1955.
How To Solve Problems. Management course for Air Force supervisors. Air Force Pamphlet No. 50:2-21, United States Government Printing Office, Washington, D.C., June, 1955.
Interpretation of the Statements of the Code for Professional Nurses. American Nurses' Association, New York, 1964.

Jourard, Sidney M.: *How Well Do You Know Your Patients?* Am. J. Nursing, 59: 11:1568, Nov., 1959.
Komorita, Nori I.: *Nursing Diagnosis.* Am. J. Nursing, 63:12:83, Dec., 1963.
Kreuter, Frances Reiter: *What Is Good Nursing Care?* Nurs. Outlook, 5:5:302, May, 1957.
Kron, Thora: *Nurses' Aides Need Clearer Directions.* Am. J. Nursing, 63:3:118, March, 1963.
Maintaining Work Flow. Social Security Administration, Division of Management, United States Government Printing Office, Washington, D.C., Jan., 1964.
Margerella, Sister Mary: *Communication: The Catalyst.* Hospital Progress, 41:5:106, May, 1960.
Mandell, Arnold J., and Mandell, Mary P.: *What Can Nursing Learn from the Behavioral Sciences?* Am. J. Nursing, 63:6:104, June, 1963.
Miller, Mary Annice: *Essentials for Self and Staff Improvement.* Am. J. Nursing, 61:11:85, Nov., 1961.
Murray, Jeanne B.: *Self-knowledge and the Nursing Interview.* Nursing Forum, 2:1:69, July, 1963.
Peplau, Heldegard E.: *Talking with Patients.* Am. J. Nursing, 60:7:964, July, 1960.
Planning and Organizing Work. Social Security Administration, Division of Management, United States Government Printing Office, Washington, D.C., Jan., 1964.
Roth, Julius A.: *How Nurses' Aides Learn their Jobs.* Am. J. Nursing, 62:8:54, Aug., 1962.
Ruhen, Olaf: *Eye Spy.* The Writer, 8 Arlington St., Boston, 76:1:9, Jan., 1963.
Schwartz, Doris R.: *Toward More Precise Evaluation of Patients' Needs.* Nurs. Outlook, 13:5:42, May, 1965.
Smith, Dorothy M.: *Myth and Method in Nursing Practice.* Am. J. Nursing, 64:2:68, Feb., 1964.
Smith, Dorothy M.: *The Nursing Team: Fact or Fancy.* Minnesota Nursing Accent (official publication of Minnesota Nurses' Association), 36:2:26, Feb., 1964.
Stephens, Gwen Jones: *The Time Factor.* Am. J. Nursing, 65:5:77, May, 1965.
The Art of Supervision. Social Security Administration, Division of Management, United States Government Printing Office, Washington, D.C., Jan. 1964.
Thomas, Betty J.: *Clues to Patients' Behavior.* Am. J. Nursing, 63:7:100, July, 1963.
Title, Monroe M.: *Public Relations Begin with the Patient.* Hospital Management, 90:3:36, Sept., 1960.
Travelbee, Joyce: *What Do We Mean by Rapport?* Am. J. Nursing, 63:2:70, Feb., 1963.
Travelbee, Joyce: *What's Wrong with Sympathy?* Am. J. Nursing, 64:1:68, Jan., 1964.
VanSant, Genee E.: *Patient's Problems Are Not Always Obvious.* Am. J. Nursing, 62:4:59, April, 1962.
VanderZanden, James W., and VanderZanden, Marion V.: *The Interview.* Nurs. Outlook, 11:10:743, Oct., 1963.
Vestal, Anne: *Problem-solving Simplified.* Hospital Progress, 41:2:78, Feb., 1960.
Wiedenbach, Ernestine: *The Helping Art of Nursing.* Am. J. Nursing, 63:11:54, Nov., 1963.
Williams, Margaret Aasterud: *The Myths and Assumptions About Team Nursing.* Nursing Forum, 3:4:61, 1964.
Winters, Margaret C., and Gilmer, Lee: *The Nurse's Judgment and the Patient's Understanding.* Am. J. Nursing, 61:12:50, Dec., 1961.
Wolff, Ilse S.: *The Educated Heart.* Am. J. Nursing, 63:4:58, April, 1963.
Wood, M. Marian: *From General Duty Nurse to Team Leader.* Am. J. Nursing, 63:1:104, Jan., 1963.
Wood, M. Marian: *Guide to Better Care—A Nursing Plan.* Am. J. Nursing, 61:12:61, Dec., 1961.

PART FOUR

The Team and Other Hospital Personnel

Wisdom is the principal thing; therefore get wisdom: and with all thy getting get understanding.

Proverbs 4:7
King James Version of the Bible

9

TEAMWORK MUST EXTEND BEYOND THE TEAM

COOPERATION BETWEEN THE TEAMS

The spirit of cooperation, while necessary among the team members themselves, must extend beyond the boundaries of the team itself. It should permeate the atmosphere of the station, the department, and the entire hospital. If the philosophy of the team plan becomes a motivating force within each team member, then its influence will grow and expand to include all personnel within the hospital.

One of the areas where cooperation is extremely important is among the teams themselves. It is very unfortunate when one team draws an invisible line, separating their patients from those of every other team, and then refuses to step over this line for any reason. Each patient is everyone's responsibility. The fact that a patient is assigned to a particular team does not mean that only members of that team are responsible for helping that patient. The activities of all hospital personnel must center around one person—the patient—and every person in every department of the hospital must share in the responsibility of his care.

The teams must work together to insure that adequate nursing care is always available for all patients on the station. While one team receives its report and assignment, the rest of the staff must assume the responsibility of caring for the patients. In addition, the time of the conference must be selected so that another team will be free to care for the patients while the one team is planning its activities.

The spirit of cooperation must extend beyond a single station. There must be teamwork among all the departments within the hospital if the aim of providing good care is to be achieved. All personnel must recognize the contribution every department makes to the welfare of the patient and be willing to work cooperatively with each department to make the services of the entire hospital available to the patient.

THE HEAD NURSE AND TEAM NURSING

The Over-all Responsibility of the Head Nurse. The head nurse is a key person not only on her station but also within the hospital. As an administrator, she is responsible for all nursing care given on her station and is concerned with the direction, supervision, and evaluation of that care. As part of this responsibility, she must coordinate not only the activities of her staff, but also all hospital services for the benefit of the patient. Since she is primarily concerned with people, she has a great responsibility in the establishment and maintenance of good human relations. The example which she sets in her day-by-day relations with her staff, with other hospital personnel, with the patients, their families, and visitors must demonstrate those attitudes and appreciations which she wants her staff to show toward others.

The head nurse must understand the aim of medical therapy for each patient and know what nursing care he needs. She must be capable of assessing the *nursing* needs of each patient. She must be capable of helping others to understand those needs and to plan how to meet the needs. In other words, every head nurse must be a master of her profession—a specialist not in nursing techniques but rather in the giving of nursing care.

The Relationships and Responsibilities of the Head Nurse in Team Nursing. Team nursing will work only to the degree to which the head nurse will allow it to function. The fact that she is efficient in managing her unit or that she insists upon her staff doing their work thoroughly does not presuppose that she can, or will, allow team nursing to function to its fullest extent. The head nurse who refuses to allow anyone else to assume additional responsibility or to make any decisions without consulting her is unable to delegate any of her authority and is, therefore, incapable of functioning within the framework of the principles of team nursing.

Good leadership by the head nurse is essential if team nursing is to be effectively practiced in her unit. She must believe wholeheartedly in the philosophy of the team plan and provide an example of democratic leadership, which can serve as a guide to the team leaders. Such a head nurse will give each team leader every opportunity for personal growth and self-expression, helping her to acquire a broader understanding of the meaning and practice of democratic leadership. She will give her the opportunity to develop those skills in the fields of administration, supervision, and teaching necessary for her to lead her team effectively. The fact that the head nurse delegates some of her duties and responsibilities to each of her team leaders does not mean that she loses prestige; rather, the need for her leadership, supervision and help increases as she guides her staff in the development of their skills and capabilities.

Team nursing allows the head nurse time to assume those responsibilities that are rightfully hers. She will be able to plan the work of her unit more efficiently and give her staff better supervision while they work. She will also be able to spend more time with the patients, determining their needs and coordinating all hospital and community services to meet these needs. She can plan her own work so that she can attend the various conferences and meetings without worrying about her unit. She can give more thought to the planning of time schedules and the writing of personnel rating reports. In other words, she has time to be a head nurse.

The assignment of personnel to each team is an important function of the head nurse, for she will need to consider the capabilities of each team leader as well as of the team members. She must insure that each team is composed of individuals who can work together harmoniously, each one complementing the abilities of the others. She must consider the members of each team when making the time schedules and must try to maintain a stable group whenever possible, thus providing a situation that can promote greater personal satisfaction for each team member and assure better continuity in patient care. She must also plan so that there will be no delay in the giving of team reports and no conflict in the times when the various teams hold their conferences. The head nurse will need to revise the membership of the team as some employees resign or rotate to other shifts and new people are employed. The orientation of recent employees is an important responsibility of the head nurse and must include an explanation of the philosophy of team nursing, the worker's contribution to the team, an introduction to all personnel on the unit, information about what her work will include, and how to do it, along with a tour to show her the physical layout of the unit.

Although the team leader may be given the responsibility of making the individual assignments to her team, the head nurse must designate the patients to be cared for by each group. She will need to revise the groups of patients as their conditions change or as some are discharged and others are admitted. Assigning an equal number of patients to each team is not always a fair distribution of responsibility. The head nurse must know the patients and their needs well enough so that she can determine the quantity of nursing care and the length of time needed to complete it. Although the number of team members will be determined in part by available personnel, all teams need not be the same size. If the physical layout of the ward is such that the patients are divided equally among the teams, the head nurse may need to revise the number on each team proportionate to the nursing care that must be given and the ability of team members to give that care.

Another major responsibility of the head nurse is that of teaching each team leader the principles of administration and supervision, which are necessary to make her leadership more effective. The head nurse should evaluate the experience and potentialities of each staff nurse. If the person is a recent graduate or a new employee with relatively little experience, the head nurse must work closely with her, helping her to plan, supervise, and evaluate the nursing care given by her team. The person who has been away from nursing for a period of time and is now returning to active duty presents an entirely different problem. In addition to becoming acquainted with her duties and responsibilities under the team plan, this person will need to learn the new treatments and techniques that have developed with the recent changes in medicine and nursing. She may have a feeling of insecurity during this learning period and needs the assurance that the head nurse is someone to whom she can go for advice and information. The part-time employee offers still another problem, since the head nurse must try to fit this individual in where she will be most useful. Because she may be unfamiliar with the patients or with recent changes in hospital policy, the head nurse must give her additional help and supervision in order to insure the giving of safe nursing care along with deriving adequate personal satisfaction from her work.

The head nurse is the person to whom the team leader should go when she encounters problems she cannot solve. These may concern the identification of patient needs and nursing problems or the evaluation of the results of nursing care. Another type of problem may be related to the organization of team activities so that the group can do its work more easily and efficiently. Errors in patient care, either of omission or commission, must be reported to the head nurse as soon as they are recognized. She is the one who must decide what action is necessary and must notify those people who are affected. A problem of public relations involving a patient, his family, or his friends must also be referred immediately to the head nurse, since this is related to public good-will toward the hospital itself. In addition, any personnel problems are of immediate concern to the head nurse, because a problem in team relationships will often give rise to other problems. The head nurse must be willing to help the team leader arrive at an acceptable solution to her problems. On occasion, she may decide to refer the matter to the departmental supervisor for further study.

Every head nurse must be a leader. She is responsible for the patient care given by her staff to each patient; she influences their attitudes toward their work and toward the patients; she acts as an example—both as a citizen and as a nurse. She can never delegate or ignore these responsibilities.

There are times when the head nurse may have to function more specifically as a team leader. She may be the only professional nurse available, or she may need to be the leader of one of the teams. Although such situations are not ideal, the head nurse who is efficient can function in both capacities for a short time. Certainly, she should never allow the giving of nursing care to lapse into the old functional method of assignment.

If you find yourself in this dual role, take a really critical look at all the things you think *you* have to do—checking and ordering supplies, checking charge slips, checking lab and x-ray slips, copying time sheets, recording TPR's, or whatever it is. Which is more important—the patient or the paper work? Oh, I know you cannot take care of the patient unless you have linen to change his bed; the patient will be upset if he doesn't get his lunch; the doctor will be unhappy if the laboratory work is not done; the nursing office will call if the time sheets do not reach there! But are *you* the only one who is intellectually capable of doing this paper work? Which requires more knowledge—giving Mrs. Brown the nursing care that she needs or copying words or figures from one piece of paper to another? Be honest with yourself. Is a nursing education necessary for all this paper work?

Your main concern should be that your team members are aware not only of *what* they should do but also of *how* they should do it. The direction and guidance that you give to your team as a whole and to each member as an individual is extremely important; therefore, you must keep them informed and expect them to report their observations to you.

The head nurse can also contribute directly to the work of the team in other ways. Since she has the over-all responsibility for the nursing care given to the patients on her station, she must be interested in the nursing care plans, must help in keeping them up to date, and must encourage the team to use them. She may wish to attend the team conferences, where she can act as a resource person, offering her suggestions concerning patient needs which she has observed. She could also offer these suggestions during the patient report. Every team leader must keep her head nurse informed about the patients and their care. In turn, the head nurse must report to each team leader any changes in treatment ordered by the doctor and give her any other information that may affect the nursing care of the patient.

Although the team leader supervises her team while they work, the head nurse supervises and evaluates the total care of all patients on her unit. If some question arises about the work of a team, the head nurse must discuss it with the team leader. The line of communication travels through the team leader to the members of the group.

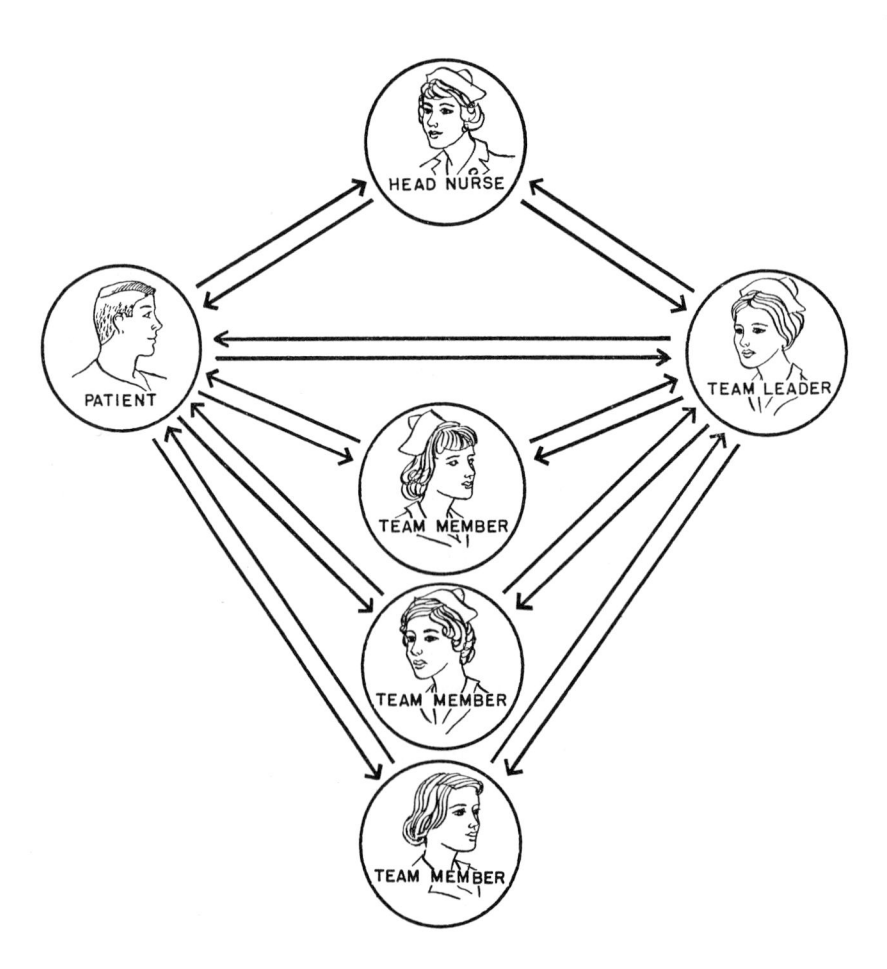

Figure 6. *Effective communication never travels in one direction only.*

THE NURSING STUDENT AND TEAM NURSING

Team nursing can be either an asset or a liability to the education of the nursing student, depending upon the interest and skill of the head nurse and the team leader in teaching the techniques of good nursing care and in giving democratic leadership. Nursing service personnel are so often concerned with the care of patients today that they forget about the person who will be giving nursing care tomorrow, or next year, or two years from now. The kind of care the patients will receive in the future can be only as good as the care the nursing student learns to give today. However, it is no longer sufficient for her to know what good nursing care is and how to give it herself; she must be given the opportunity to learn and to practice those skills needed in directing and supervising others in the giving of total patient care. She must recognize the importance of good human relations and learn to work cooperatively with others in meeting the nursing care needs of the patients.

Early Experience in Team Nursing. The nursing student should become a member of a nursing team from the beginning of her clinical experience; in this way, she can learn through observation and personal experience how the team functions. She can see teamwork in action and learn the importance of cooperation in the giving of good patient care. As she attends the team conferences, she can learn how patient-centered care is planned, and as she receives a report and listens to the explanation of the individual assignments to the team members, she will realize how that plan is carried out.

School policies must be followed when planning the student's assignment; however, it may be made out by the head nurse or the team leader in cooperation with the clinical instructor. Every assignment must be planned on the basis of the learning needs of the student. Early in her experience she needs to gain skill in the performance of nursing techniques and in the actual planning, giving, and evaluating of the patient's care. As she carries out this assignment, the team leader should be willing to offer assistance whenever the student shows a need. Although the student is concerned with giving complete care to some patients, she must also be made to feel that she is a part of the team, perhaps by being assigned to assist with certain parts of a patient's care which an aide cannot perform. Thus, the student begins to learn how to work with people and how to coordinate the work of several persons to provide individualized patient care.

Since the team leader is responsible for the nursing care given by her team, she will want to supervise and help the student in the giving of that care. However, she shares this responsibility with the head nurse and the clinical instructor, for all three must work together to plan a good learning experience for the student and to help her gain the necessary knowledge, understanding, and skills required by the professional nurse.

The Nursing Student as Team Leader. As the nursing student becomes more skillful in performing the required techniques, in understanding the needs of her patients, and in helping them to solve their problems, she should learn how to guide and direct others in giving patient-centered care. This may be done by giving her the opportunity to act as team leader.

If the student is to acquire acceptable attitudes toward and appreciations of her professional responsibilities as a leader, her experience as a team leader must be carefully planned and closely supervised. She must recognize the importance of human relations and learn to apply the principles of democratic leadership in all her team relations. She must be helped and encouraged to increase her skills in planning and evaluating patient-centered care, in solving nursing problems, and in directing and supervising the work of others. She must learn what team leadership requires and how to effectively meet her responsibilities toward her patients, the members of her team, and herself.

Throughout the entire clinical experience of the nursing student, emphasis must be placed on methods of individualizing the nursing care of each patient. The head nurse and the team leader must be especially careful to plan her assignments in such a way that the idea of performing nursing techniques on a functional basis is minimized and, instead, the part each has in the total care of the patient is emphasized. Especially when acting as team leader, the nursing student must be made to realize that her responsibility to her team and to her patients goes beyond the mere giving of treatments and medications and doing the necessary recording on the patient's chart. However, if she is to realize and appreciate fully the scope of this responsibility, she must have been brought up in an atmosphere of teamwork from the very beginning of her clinical experience and have had the opportunity to observe other team leaders as they effectively put into practice the principles of team leadership.

THE CLINICAL INSTRUCTOR AND TEAM NURSING

Cooperation between the team leader, head nurse, and clinical instructor is absolutely essential in order to provide the nursing student with a good learning experience and adequate supervision. Each one has an important contribution to make to the education of the student, but, if an atmosphere conducive to learning is to be provided, each must understand the aims and problems of the others. It is important that both the head nurse and the team leader remember that the nursing student is present on the ward primarily for the purpose of learning and only secondarily for service. Until they gain an appreciation of this fact, the nursing student will fail to gain a complete experience either in the giving of nursing care or in an appreciation of her responsibilities as a professional nurse. Every nursing student must be provided with a good clinical education if the head nurse is to have, in the future, well-prepared nurses who will be able to give good nursing care and to assume the responsibilities required of them. The student's attitudes about what her role in nursing is, and how to fulfill it, are being formed by her experiences today.

The clinical instructor should strive to interpret the aims of nursing education to the head nurse and team leader and to help them in planning the student's experience so that these aims can be met. On the other hand, the clinical instructor must realize that the immediate care of the patient is of primary concern to the nursing service personnel; therefore, she must be willing to work with these people in supervising and guiding the student.

Especially in planning the assignment for the nursing student, the clinical instructor, the head nurse, and the team leader must work closely together. The activities of the station will become disorganized unless this assignment is planned well and all three know exactly what the student is to do. More important, the patient and part of his care may be neglected unless all are kept informed. However, the head nurse and team leader must remember that occasionally a student's assignment may need to be changed on short notice in order to provide her with experience in an unforeseen learning situation which arises. On the other hand, the clinical instructor should try to look ahead so that such changes are made with a minimum amount of confusion.

The clinical instructor should be an ex-officio member of any team of which the student is a member, especially if the student is acting as team leader. She will need to work with the student in identifying the needs of the patients and in planning their care. She will also need to help her to acquire the necessary skills to effectively lead the team conference, to supervise her team in giving the patient care as indicated on the care plan, and finally, in evaluating the effectiveness of that care and of her own leadership.

THE NURSING SUPERVISOR AND TEAM NURSING

The role of the nursing supervisor has been much discussed in professional circles, with the result that there seems to be a question concerning just what her role should be. Since the supervisor is usually concerned with an entire department, made up of several nursing units, she has the opportunity to get a broader picture of how the nursing needs of the patients are being met, how the various members of her department are working together, and how her department can work more cooperatively with the other departments in the hospital. Because of her additional skills and experience, she should be able to help the head nurses in solving the problems arising on the various stations. She can also help in establishing and keeping open the lines of communication between hospital administration and the head nurses.

She can also play an important part in the functioning of team nursing, first, by helping the head nurses to develop a better understanding of the team members' place in the team plan and, secondly, by helping them to become more democratic in their leadership. The nursing supervisor must demonstrate her interest in the effective functioning of the team members. She is in an excellent position to interpret the aims of the team plan to hospital administration and to explain how it can be made to work more efficiently.

Perhaps one of her biggest opportunities for increasing the scope of her supervision is in the field of research. Whenever nursing service problems are referred to her, she should try to plan cooperatively with the personnel involved so that a better method of giving nursing care may be discovered through the solution of these problems. She should always be on the lookout for more efficient work methods, either by revising established procedures or by using different equipment.

THE LICENSED PRACTICAL NURSE AND TEAM NURSING

The licensed practical nurse (L.P.N.) or licensed vocational nurse (L.V.N.) is trained to care for patients under the direction and supervision of a registered nurse or a physician. The L.P.N. may take care of patients in "simple nursing situations" or assist the registered nurse in the care of those patients who present "complex nursing situations."* There is, however, wide variation in the interpretation of the functions of the L.P.N. There is also no standard definition of the terms, *direction* and *supervision,* although *direction* implies distance whereas *supervision* indicates closer observation and help by a professional nurse or a doctor.

With the growth and increased complexity of medical practice, the registered nurse has assumed more and more of the therapeutic

---

Statement of Functions of the Licensed Practical Nurse. American Nurses Association, 1964.

techniques delegated to nursing by the doctor. The registered nurse, in turn, has delegated some of her duties to other workers. It is ironic that the professional nurse has given away her birthright—the giving of direct nursing care—to the L.P.N. and the ancillary worker and has chosen instead a secondary role—the performance of therapeutic techniques as directed by the physician.

By virtue of her education the registered nurse is supposed to possess the ability to judge and make decisions about the nursing care of her patients. This ability, which sets her apart from the practical nurse, is necessary in the making of a nursing diagnosis and the decision on the appropriate nursing intervention measures.

Because the L.P.N. does not have the educational background that would enable her to make qualified judgments and decisions about patient care, she cannot function as team leader; however, the L.P.N. can be a great asset in team nursing for, with the guidance and supervision of the professional nurse, the L.P.N. can function in her true role of assisting in the care of the patients. Today's L.P.N. has the skill to perform many of the therapeutic techniques delegated by the doctor to nursing, but she needs help from the team leader to adapt the procedures to the individual patient. Furthermore, because the L.P.N. spends much of her time with the patient and because she does have a better understanding of patient care than the nurses' aide, she can contribute much information during the team conference to help define and evaluate the nursing care of each patient.

The team leader must learn how to use the L.P.N.'s skills without causing her to exceed the limits imposed by the description of her job. On the other hand, the team leader must know the ability of each L.P.N. because she may not be capable of performing certain techniques even though the hospital policy may allow it. In addition, the team leader must determine when she may give direction only and when she must give supervision so that the patient will receive safe and effective care at all times.

The team plan can be constantly expanded as the personnel realize to a greater extent what can be accomplished through teamwork and make use of every opportunity for personal growth. Continuous in-service programs for the professional nurses must be carried on to help them increase their understanding of team nursing and ways of applying its principles to their own situation. The training of the nonprofessional personnel cannot be carried on solely by the head nurse and the team leader. A program of instruction is necessary for these people, especially for those recently employed, although the head nurse and team leader will both need to reinforce and enlarge upon the teaching given in this program.

The fullest expression of the principles of team nursing will not be achieved in one month, one year, or even two years, for, as the team members grow in wisdom and understanding, so will also their concept of the work of the nursing team continue to grow. Yet team leadership will always remain a challenge to the professional nurse, and her democratic leadership will always be the key to a successful nursing team.

STUDY QUESTIONS

1. If you are associated with a school of nursing, what are its objectives? What are the means used to achieve these aims and objectives? What are the objectives of the nursing service department? Discuss the relationships between the objectives of these two departments.

2. How could cooperation be increased between two or more departments in your hospital?

3. Discuss the responsibilities of the head nurse in your hospital for aiding in the education of the nursing student.

4. Discuss the areas in which the team leader may help in the education of the nursing student.

5. List as many specific duties as you can that are now performed by the head nurse. Analyze each one. Which ones could be performed by someone else? Which ones must remain the responsibility of the head nurse?

6. Give specific suggestions as to how the head nurse can participate in team activities.

7. Give specific suggestions as to how the supervisor can participate in team activities.

8. Do you believe that the concept of the team plan can ever be practiced to its fullest extent? Give your reasons.

PART FOUR BIBLIOGRAPHY

Books

Barrett, Jean: *The Head Nurse.* Appleton-Century-Crofts, Inc., New York, 1963.
Lambertsen, Eleanor: *Nursing Team—Organization and Functioning.* Published for the Division of Nursing Education, Bureau of Publications, Teacher's College, Columbia University, New York, 1953.
Newcomb, Dorothy Perkins: *The Team Plan. A Manual for Nursing Service Administrators.* G. P. Putnam's Sons, Inc., New York, 1953.

Journals

Auxiliary Personnel in Nursing Service. Am. J. Nursing, 62:7:22, July, 1962.
Barrett, Jean: *The Head Nurse's Changing Role.* Nurs. Outlook, 11:11:80, Nov., 1963.
Barrett, Kathleen M.: *The Student as Team Leader.* Am. J. Nursing, 50:8:498, Aug., 1950.
Brackett, Mary E., and Fogt, Joan R.: *Is Comprehensive Nursing Care a Realistic Goal?* Nurs. Outlook, 9:7:402, July, 1961.

Brooks, Ethel A.: *Team Nursing—1961.* Am. J. Nursing, April, 1961.
Brown, William King: *An Administrator's View of the Head Nurse's Work.* Nurs. Outlook, 11:11:798, Nov., 1963.
Coletti, Angela C.: *The Head Nurse Is a Manager.* Hospital Progress, 41:3:100, March, 1960.
Cook, Billie Jo McCullars, and Festog, Eleanor I.: *Talk About Team Nursing.* Am. J. Nursing, 63:11:93, Nov., 1963.
Doan, Joseph: *Ten Attributes of a Good Administrator.* Modern Hospital, 60:5:61, May, 1945.
Dudley, Martha: *The Head Nurse's Dilemma.* RN, 25:7:41, July, 1962.
Hannan, A., Judy, E., and Colosanti, E.: *The Head Nurse Functions in the Team Plan.* Am. J. Nursing, 51:8:500, Aug., 1951.
Jennings, Muriel: *On-the-Job Counseling.* Am. J. Nursing, 61:3:67, March, 1961.
Leino, Amelia: *Organizing the Nursing Team.* Am. J. Nursing, 51:11:665, Nov., 1951.
Merton, Robert K.: *Relations Between Registered Nurses and Licensed Practical Nurses.* Am. J. Nursing, 62:10:70, Oct., 1962.
Miller, Mary Annice: *Essentials for Self and Staff Improvement.* Am. J. Nursing, 61:11:85, Nov., 1961.
Muller, Theresa G.: *The Head Nurse as a Teacher.* Nurs. Outlook, 11:1:46, Jan., 1963.
Osborne, Estelle: *Teamwork.* Am. J. Nursing, 50:6:367, June, 1950.
Russo, Michael: *Practical Nursing and the Team Approach.* Practical Nursing Digest, 10:5:133, Nov., 1963.
Scott, Jessie M.: *Seeing Nursing Activities as They Are.* Am. J. Nursing, 62:11:70, Nov., 1962.
Shepardson, Jeanette: *Developing a Job Description.* Am. J. Nursing, 62:4:62, April, 1962.
Sister Juliana: *Team Nursing: Student Style.* Hospital Progress, 45(7):104, July, 1964.

Index

Abilities, individual, 25-27, 33
Abstract words, 47, 72
Administration, defined, 30, 87
 economy in, 34
 leadership and, 30-35
 principles of, 30-35
 reports vital to, 34, 68
 supervision and, 35, 37, 98
Aims, of hospital, 3, 30-31
 of departments in, 3, 31
 of nursing care, 127, 134, 141-142
 of team nursing, 12, 35, 57, 66, 126, 132
Anecdotal notes, 107-110
Assignment(s), by head nurse, 157-158
 individual, 73-77
 legal aspects of, 87-90
 methods of making, 12, 71-78, 81-83, 88-89, 143
 preceded by orientation, 67-68
 preceded by reports, 71
Attitudes, 24-25

Basic needs of people, 19-23, 58
Belong, need to, 20-21

Challenge of team leadership, 13, 166
Changes affecting nursing, 6-10
Clinical instructor, team nursing and, 162-163
Communication, 43-49, 72, 93-95
 as aid to cooperation, 66-67
 barriers to, 44-48
 defined, 44
 during team conference, 123-129
 human relations and, 110-113
 in supervision, 90

Communication (*Continued*)
 lines of, 31-32, 160, 164
 listening as part of, 44-49, 101-102
 methods used, 44-49
  in nursing care plan, 132-133
  in reports, 68-71
  when giving directions, 41, 72-77, 89
 rumors and, 49
 understanding as part of, 45-46
Comprehensive nursing, defined, 4
Conference, team, 117-131, 142, 143
 conducting, 123-129
 head nurse in, 159
Cooperation, aided by communication, 66-67
 effect of, on team nursing, 155-156
 in administration, 33
 in nursing care, 118-119
 in team leadership, 42
 in team nursing, 39, 160
 methods of obtaining, 29-30, 33, 42, 60, 66-67, 77, 99, 101, 111-113, 117-119, 129
Coordination, in administration, 33
 in team leadership, 42-43, 71-72, 118
Counseling, as aid to improvement, 107-110
Creative leadership, 29
 examples of, 36, 38-40, 60, 77

Definitions, administration, 30
 communication, 44
 comprehensive nursing care, 4
 direction, 89, 164
 guidance, 41
 individualized patient care, 4
 leadership, 28
 learning, 91

169

Definitions (*Continued*)
  nursing care, 4, 5, 33
  nursing operation, 4
  orientation, 67
  patient-centered care, 4
  planning, 57–58
  supervision, 35–36, 86–87, 89, 164
  team, 38
  total patient care, 4
  wisdom, 91
Delegation of responsibility, 31–32, 63–65, 75, 88–89, 165
Differences, individual, 25–27, 33, 58, 74
Directions, giving, 41, 72–77, 89
Directive leadership, 29
  examples of, 36, 38–40, 60, 77

Economic conditions, changes in, 7–8
Economy in administration, 34
Education, nursing, changes in, 8–10
Emotions, 23, 26
Evaluation, after observation, 76–77, 104–105, 106–110
  legal aspects, 89
  of patient care, 133
  of team, 103–110, 127, 144
  of team leadership, 43, 50–51, 104, 106, 148–149
  of work organization, 80

Guidance, as aid to improvement, 107–110
  defined, 41
  in team leadership, 41–42

Head nurse, in team nursing, 156–160
  responsibilities, 12, 32, 81, 88, 113, 156, 157
Hospital(s), aims of, 3, 30–31
  changes in, 7
  economy in, 31
  organization of, 31
Human relations, 33, 36, 104, 110–113, 156, 161

Individual assignments, 73–77
Individual differences, 25–27, 33, 58, 74
Individual patient care, defined, 4
  planning for, 117–118, 133–148
  providing, 74–75
In-service education, 165–166

Instructor, clinical, team nursing and, 162–163
Interpersonal relationships, 33, 104, 110–113
Interview of patient, 135

Job descriptions, 58, 90

Knowledge, 26, 57–58, 73, 91

Leadership, 28–51
  administration and, 30–35
  creative, 29, 36, 38–40, 60, 77
  defined, 28–30
  democratic, 13, 29, 36, 38–40, 60, 77
  directive, 29, 36, 38–40, 60, 77
  qualities for, 49–51, 91
  results of, 30
  supervision and, 35–37
  types of, 29–30, 33
Learning, ability for, 25
  defined, 86–87, 91
  results of, 92
Legal aspects of team nursing, 87–90
Licensed practical nurse, 12, 38, 89, 90
  team nursing and, 164–165
Listening, 44, 45–46, 48, 101–102

Manual dexterity, 26
Medicine, changes in, 6
Methods, of communication, 43–45, 48–49
  of giving directions, 72–77
  of giving reports, 68–71
  of making assignments, 72–77
  of observing, 98–106
  of organizing work, 57–65
  of planning nursing care, 133–145
  of supervising, 86–116

Need(s), basic, 19–23
  for recognition, 19
  for security, 23, 58
  for stimulation, 23, 58
  to belong, 20–21
Negligence, 90
Nurse, clinician, 10
  duties and responsibilities, 9–12, 30, 38, 164–165

INDEX

Nurse (*Continued*)
  head, in team nursing, 156-160
    responsibilities, 12, 32, 81, 88, 113, 156, 157
  licensed practical, 12, 38, 89, 90
    team nursing and, 164-165
  technician, 10
Nurses' aide, 11, 68, 82, 88, 90
Nursing, changes affecting, 6-10
  diagnosis, 9, 88, 117-118
  comprehensive, 4
  problems confronting, 10-13
Nursing care, aim of, 127, 134, 141-142
  components of, 133-142
  defined, 3-6, 62-63, 133
  legal aspects of planning, 88
  objectives of, 134, 141-142
  plans for, 9, 12, 74, 88, 117-118, 127, 132-148
Nursing education, changes in, 8-10
Nursing students, team nursing and, 78, 90, 161-162

Objectives of nursing care, 134, 141-142
Observation, in team leadership, 43, 45, 76
  techniques of, 98-106
Organization of work, 31-32, 57-85
  evaluation, 80
Organizational chart, 31
Orientation, 67-68, 144
  defined, 67

Participation, in team conference, 124-125
  in team leadership, 38, 42
Part-time personnel, 71, 81-82, 156
Patient, interview of, 135
Patient-centered care, defined, 4
  planning for, 9, 12, 88, 117-118, 132, 133-148
  providing, 74-75
People, attitudes of, 24
  basic needs, 19-23, 58
  differences of, 25-27, 33, 58, 74
  emotions of, 23
Personnel, number of, 12, 32
Persuasion, 48-49
Planning, administration and, 31-34
  defined, 57-58
  for the team conference, 119-123
  in team leadership, 41
  in work organization, 57-65, 78-79
  nursing care, 133-145
Principles, of administration, 38-43
  of team leadership, 38-43

Problems, confronting nursing, 10-12
  solving of, 58-62
    team nursing as a solution to, 12-13

Qualities of a leader, 49-51, 91

Recognition, need for, 19
Reports, illustration of in problem-solving, 60-62
  in administration, 34-35, 68
  legal aspects of, 89
  method of giving, 68-71, 80-81
  nursing care plan and, 143
  use of, in giving assignments, 71
Responsibility, delegation of, 31-32, 63-65, 75, 88-89, 165
Results of leadership, 30
  of learning, 92
Rumors, 49

Scientific thinking, 58-62
Security, need for, 23, 58
Senses, use in observation, 98-102
Social conditions, changes in, 7-8
Solving problems, methods of, 58-62
Stimulation, need for, 23, 58
Students, nursing, team nursing and, 78, 90, 161-162
Supervision, as key to team leadership, 86-87, 114
  by professional nurse, 12-13, 89
  defined, 35-36, 37, 87, 89
  evaluation of, 106, 144
  human relations and, 33, 36, 104, 110-113
  legal aspects of, 87-90
  methods of, 86-116
  need for, 86-87, 97-98
  nursing care plans and, 133, 144
  purposes of, 36-37
  teaching and, 91-96
  types of, 35-36
Supervisor, team nursing and, 163-164

Teaching, during team conference, 125-127
  fallacies concerning, 91-92
  steps used in, 92-96
  supervision and, 91-96
Team, assignments, 12, 71-78, 81-83, 88-89, 143

Team (*Continued*)
  conference, 12, 117–131, 142, 143
  defined, 38
  evaluation of, 103–106, 107–110, 127
  leader of, activities, 12–13, 31–35, 40–43, 48–49, 82–83, 86–87, 121–122, 142, 148–149, 160, 161 (57–149)
  report, 68–71, 80–81
  spirit, 66–67, 117–119
  supervision of, 86–116, 144
  understanding, need for, 66–67, 70, 76, 118, 133
Team leadership, challenge of, 13, 166
  evaluation of, 106, 144, 148–149
  head nurse and, 156–160
  in team conference, 117–131
  supervision and, 89, 90–91
  teamwork and, 38
  techniques, 40–43, 48–49, 57–149
Team nursing, aim of, 12, 35, 57, 66, 86, 126
  as aid in solving problems, 12–13
  clinical instructor and, 160–161
  head nurse and, 156–160
  leadership techniques in, 38–43, 48–49, 57–149

Team nursing (*Continued*)
  licensed practical nurse and, 164–165
  nursing student and, 161–162
  nursing supervisor and, 159, 161–162
  twenty-four hour use of, 82, 115, 119–120
  type of leadership in, 38–40
Teamwork, 38, 66–67
Thinking, problem solving and, 58–60
Total patient care, defined, 4

Understanding, barriers to, 46–48
  communication and, 45–48
  defined, 91
  need for, 21–22, 44–49, 66–67, 70, 76, 118
Use of senses in observation, 98–102

Wisdom, defined, 91
Words, abstract, 47, 72
Work organization, 31–32, 57–85
  evaluation of, 79–80
Work plans, 63–65, 78